1987

Marketing
Religious
Health Care

Robin Scott MacStravic

The Catholic Health Association of the United States
St. Louis, MO

Library of Congress Cataloging-in-Publication Data

MacStravic, Robin E. Scott.
   Marketing religious health care.

   Includes index.
   1. Religious health facilities — Marketing.
I. Catholic Health Association of the United States.
II. Title. [DNLM: 1. Delivery of Health Care — United States. 2. Marketing
of Health Services. 3. Religion and Medicine. W 74 M479m]
RA975.R44M33 1987 362.1'068'8   86-29937
ISBN 0-87125-121-3

TABLE OF CONTENTS

Introduction

This book is for everyone in religious health care organizations who is involved in or concerned about attracting and satisfying those who use their services. It addresses how to use marketing principles and techniques in hospitals, nursing homes, and any other facilities that religious communities, congregations, and organizations sponsor. It is written out of a strong conviction that marketing is too important for marketing staff persons alone to handle. Only when all members of the organization understand and appreciate their roles in attracting and satisfying patients can they contribute optimally to their institution's success and survival.

This book is also written out of the strong conviction that although health care organizations must adopt businesslike ways of thinking and operating in today's competitive environment, health care delivery is much more than a business. Health care providers have a far greater obligation to those they serve than do commercial purveyors of goods and services. They must somehow adopt the techniques of business without adopting its mercantile values. A marketing text can describe little that religious health care organizations are uniquely capable of doing. Such organizations, however, may be uniquely willing to perform certain tasks that have distinct marketing value.

Religious health care organizations should have the distinct marketing advantage of strong and lasting values that all its members can share and practice. The most successful business organizations often prosper under the strong leadership of a single individual who is able to convey and embody a set of values that successfully motivates the organization's members. Too often, that set of values and its motivating effect are lost with the founder's death or retirement. Religious organizations have centuries of history and tradition and a permanent basis for their values that should prevent such a loss.

The values of service to fellow human beings, respect for each person's dignity and worth, and caring for those less fortunate should have distinct marketing impact in health care. The more clearly and strongly health care facilities express these values through day-to-day operation, the more successful they are likely to be in marketing as well as mission. Marketing is a pragmatic discipline that individuals and organizations with widely varying values can use. The fact that marketing can give religious health care organizations a competitive advantage is a function of human nature more than marketing.

Patients often seek health care because of anxiety, hope, despair, guilt, and loneliness. Religious health care organizations have something to offer in such circumstances that others lack. The key to successful marketing as well as to mission achievement is fulfilling the religious promise, living out religious values in day-to-day operations, and responding to the full scope of human needs. This book offers guidance and suggestions on how to express values in marketing strategies and tactics to promote health care facilities' success and survival.

At its worst, marketing can be used to exploit human needs. In the long run, however, marketing succeeds only by identifying and responding to human needs better. It calls on organizations to consistently improve how they address human needs and to do this better than competing organizations. Given the range and complexity of human needs, no one model of operation is bound to succeed. Marketing is a way of constantly striving to do better, both better than yesterday and better than the competition. Such striving should be familiar to religious organizations.

The Golden Rule is probably the best expression of how to succeed in marketing services, since it summarizes religious values regarding human interactions. It would be foolish to claim that religious organizations are guaranteed a marketing advantage, but one is available to them if they can live out their values in service transactions. This book offers some practical models and specific suggestions on how organizations might translate such values into marketing as well as mission success.

There may be many who see a significant and perilous conflict between the spiritual values that motivate religious health care organizations and the commercial values associated with marketing. Marketing has no values of its own; only those who employ its concepts and techniques need be bound by values. On the other hand, the more I learn from market research, the more I become convinced that what people want from marketers is what religious values tell us we should give them.

Religious values call for respecting the dignity and worth of every individual. It should come as no surprise that almost all individuals want respect for dignity and worth. Religious values call for recognizing and responding to the full scope of human needs, the psychological, social, economic, and spiritual as well as physical. Market research consistently shows that people want the full scope of their needs recognized, and that they respond favorably to organizations that do so.

Our values call on us to promote truly informed consent, participation in making decisions, the right to make choices. Patients and their families, as shown in marketing research results, are increasingly calling for us to give them choices, to respect their need and desire for information and participation. We have professional knowledge and skills that enable us to serve patients in ways they are unable to do for themselves. Marketing demands that we serve others as they wish to be served, in addition to serving them as we wish to.

The Golden Rule asks us to do unto others as we would have them do unto us. Marketing only slightly paraphrases this rule and asks that we do unto others as they would have us do unto them. What makes marketing work is its ability to learn what people need, want, and wish for, then figure out how to deliver it to them, then tell them about it in a persuasive manner. We may set out to serve others in terms of what we think they need or should want. Marketing merely insists that we also take into account what they think they want.

In health care, we have always had to deal with the competition and occasional conflict between professional quality of care and management quality of operation. Responding to the needs of each patient, doing what is best for each individual will inevitably run counter to pursuing high levels of productivity and efficiency, at least some of the time.

Marketing adds a third concern, for customer quality. A useful rule of thumb in services marketing is to look for opportunities to respond to peculiar needs, wants, and desires of individuals, as well as offer uniformly good customer experiences. It is common "boilerplate" in customer relations to suggest something like: "If there is anything we can do to make your (trip, stay, etc.) more enjoyable, please let us know." We know this isn't meant to be taken seriously, and most of us rarely if ever come up with any request.

In health care marketing, especially in extended patient care encounters or relationships, it would be wise to make this cliché mean something. My research consistently suggests that the patient that has one off-the-wall wish, is encouraged to request it and has it granted, is likely to be not only satisfied but delighted by the experience. Doing so will always require bending standard procedures and thereby threatening efficiency. In most cases, however, it will be worth it.

Marketing, in the sense of promoting the attraction and satisfaction of as many customers as possible, promises rewards to everyone associated with the organization. Satisfying patients promotes physician and employee satisfaction; it enhances morale as well as financial success. Marketing offers us opportunities to do better in all aspects of our mission as well as to enhance the probability of surviving and financing our charitable mission.

Chapter 1 defines marketing and breaks it down into five basic components. Each marketing organization must work at (1) discovering, (2) deciding, (3) designing, (4) delivering, and (5) describing health care experiences, both for the immediate consumers of such services (patients, residents, clients, guests) and for all others involved in health care. This chapter summarizes the marketing process and is aimed at every member of the health care organization.

Chapter 2 briefly discusses the marketing intelligence function: understanding consumers and other decision makers and their knowledge, beliefs, attitudes, and behavior. The discovery step in marketing serves as a basis for all subsequent effort. It identifies market and consumer behavior dynamics, intangible perceptions and tangible causes, and competitive positions in the market and in individual's minds. It strives to understand human needs and available responses as a basis for deciding, designing, delivering, and describing better ways to respond to them. This chapter is targeted at everyone involved in designing, generating, or using marketing research within the organization.

Chapter 3 examines the strategic marketing function: deciding who the organization should strive to serve, what services it should offer, and how it can succeed in its mission as well as promote its survival. This step addresses questions of how, where, and when to use marketing techniques and for what purposes. This chapter is aimed at everyone who participates in deciding on the organization's overall mission and in determining how best to implement it.

Chapter 4 examines the tactical marketing function: designing how to implement specific services and marketing initiatives. It focuses on how to create service experiences that are optimally attractive and satisfying to their users and other decision makers, as well as supportive of the organization's mission and survival. The chapter is targeted at everyone who participates in determining how the organization's mission will be translated into operation.

Chapter 5 discusses the internal marketing function: delivering what has been decided and designed. It focuses on managing human resources to deliver the intended health care experience optimally. This chapter is aimed at every manager, supervisor, and employee that contributes to the health care experience.

Chapter 6 examines the marketing communications function: describing what has been designed and is being delivered to promote the organization and satisfy service users and other decision makers. It uses a positioning model, which focuses on how persons "place" competing services and providers using judgments that affect their choices. This chapter is intended for everyone involved in designing, testing, and evaluating marketing communications.

Chapter 7 discusses the marketing evaluation function: discovering what has happened, what can be attributed to specific marketing efforts, and deciding how valuable the effects are to the organization. Each step in the marketing process should be evaluated, in addition to assessing the total effort. This chapter is aimed at everyone who participates in determining a marketing effort's effectiveness and efficiency.

Chapter 8 offers suggestions on how organizations can address religious values and marketing realities simultaneously in relations with health care consumers. It describes how each marketing function is used in a strategy based on evidence of excellence. By addressing what is important to both customers and the organization, marketing through evidence can promote mission achievement as well as marketing success and the organization's survival.

Chapter 9 describes a specific marketing strategy that religious health care organizations might consider using. Striving to be and become known as *the* personal provider of health services, the organization with a distinct and positive personality, should follow the organization's values closely and have significant marketing benefit. This chapter is aimed at all personnel who participate in marketing their organization's services.

1. The Marketing Challenge

Most discussions of marketing health care begin with a definition of marketing to counter some common misconceptions. Whether such misconceptions still exist after so many careful definitions is hard to determine. To be safe, and to provide a framework for subsequent discussion, a definition may be helpful.

The official definition of marketing comes from the American Marketing Association, which adopted it in 1985 to replace an earlier version adopted in 1960. It states that: "Marketing is the process of planning and executing the conception, pricing, promotion, and distribution of ideas, goods, and services to create exchanges that satisfy individual and organizational objectives."[1] This is easily the broadest definition of what marketing is supposed to mean, a definition far broader than the ideas and activities most persons associate with the term.

The definition points out that marketing includes both planning and executing, both thinking and doing. It is not a staff function but necessarily crosses over into a health care organization's entire operation. Marketing covers all aspects of designing programs, including pricing and promoting them. It can be used with goods and services, but also with ideas. Marketers would be happy to advise churches on how to market religion. Marketing focuses on a simple idea: the concept of exchange. If consumers think they will be better off by buying a particular good, using a particular service, or adopting a particular behavior, they will usually do so. Marketing's challenge is to convince persons that they will be better off, make them better off, and ensure that the organization will be better off as a result of these behavioral responses.

One can review marketing as involving five categories of activities, the "five Ds": discovering, deciding, designing, delivering, and describing. These activities interact with each other and are constantly repeated in any organization engaged in marketing. Their collective purpose is to bring about behavior patterns in the market that support the organization's mission and contribute to its vitality. Marketing is a form of behavioral engineering, a practical application of the principles, knowledge, and techniques of the behavioral sciences to understand, predict, and influence people's behavior.

The Five Ds

Discovering represents the essential starting point in any marketing effort. The first of the Ds includes all activities that lead to a better understanding of the organization, its markets, its environment, and its competition. Initially, research and analysis focus on discovering enough so the individual or organization can move on to the next steps of deciding, designing, delivering, and describing. Each step relies on and is influenced by what the first step reveals. Discovering also begins the cycle again as research is used to identify and evaluate the effects, if any, of specific marketing tactics and total marketing strategies.

Deciding represents strategic marketing: the planning of the organization's future. The organization reconsiders and redefines its mission and determines (1) those consumers it intends to serve, (2) what particular set of services it intends to offer, and (3) how it will survive in a competitive and often hostile environment. Strategic decisions form the basis for designing and delivering services at a tactical level and for describing what the health care organization offers effectively and efficiently.

Designing combines the insights gained through discovering with the choices made in deciding to develop or modify services and patient experience in order to promote achievement of organizational goals and objectives. After marketers make strategic decisions regarding the entire health care organization and its programs, they make design choices with respect to individual programs and specific aspects of the patient experience. Designing focuses on making the patient experience, as well as that of the family, physician, employee, volunteer, and donor, as attractive and satisfying as possible, while furthering organizational mission and vitality.

Delivering represents the operations side of marketing: making sure that the decided and designed programs are put into practice. Deciding represents strategic marketing and designing is tactical marketing, whereas delivering is internal marketing. It includes all steps necessary to obtain, organize, direct, and control resources in order to attract and satisfy markets and ensure the quality, efficiency, and cost effectiveness of operations. This is where marketing gives way to management and supervision, but it is the most critical of the marketing activities.

Describing takes what the organization has discovered and designed plus what it intends to deliver or is delivering and communicates to intended markets so as to promote attraction and satisfaction. It is the external marketing function: talking about what it is doing. Describing alone rarely achieves the desired effect on market behavior; design and delivery are necessary allies. At the same time, unless the organization describes to prospects what it has designed and is delivering, the effects are likely to be wasted or at least limited. Rather than "hiding one's light under a bushel basket," religious health care organizations should have no doubts about the value of describing what they offer to interested parties.

Marketing Language

It is traditional in health care to refer to those persons served as *patients* (in hospitals and clinics) or *residents* (in nursing homes) and occasionally as *clients* (for social welfare services). The traditional marketing term, *consumer,* does not apply particularly well, especially since it pertains to products more than services. In health care marketing, it is essential first to distinguish between those who are served directly (patients, residents, or clients) and those who actually decide whether and from whom to seek particular services.

Traditionally, in hospitals one thinks of the physician as the basic decision maker. In nursing home marketing, an elderly parent's children, often a daughter or daughter-in-law, are principal decision makers. Increasingly, persons are making their own health care choices, "shopping" for specialists and "self-referring" to sports medicine, alcohol treatment, plastic surgery, and other services. To clarify whether and where discussions refer to the users of services or to decision makers, this book uses an arbitrary language convention. The term *guest* refers here to patients, residents, and other direct recipients of service, whereas the term *customer* applies to all decision makers, including guests. The term *prospect* refers to potential customers and guests.

The word guest is used to suggest that health care providers have special obligations to those they serve, far beyond what is typical for retail sales organizations, for example. Customer is used to remind health providers that they are dealing with persons who can make choices, who have the right to demand service, and who will go elsewhere for it if they wish. Religious health care organizations have to be able to manage their affairs in a businesslike manner in order to survive and continue their missions. They are more than businesses, however; they are missions and services to the community. Marketing carries with it many business-like and even warlike concepts and language,[2] but it can serve health care as long as providers do not lose sight of the obligations that make them more than businesses.

Attraction and Satisfaction

All five basic marketing steps focus on the essential marketing purpose of attracting prospects and satisfying customers and guests. This also applies to any other groups of people, or *publics* in marketing jargon, whose behavior can contribute to the health care organization's mission achievements and vitality. All marketing activities are based first on what such publics need, want, desire, and demand. Discovering tries to understand publics; deciding chooses what to do about them; designing develops ways to respond to them; delivering builds relationships with them; and describing talks to them. All five activities focus heavily on factors outside the organization, on what publics want from the organization.

Most health care organizations are interested in attracting new guests, physicians, employees, volunteers, donors, employers, or other "customers." Often, the principal justification for engaging in a new or expanded marketing effort is the desire to increase business. Whether mission or survival demands it, bringing in new customers is probably the first goal of marketing.

Health care organizations should deem satisfying (or preferably pleasing and delighting) present customers at least as important as attracting new ones. Organizations are unlikely to survive or achieve their missions by attraction alone. Physicians, employees, and volunteers should remain members of the organization; patients, donors, and employers should continue in an active and lasting relationship with the organization. It takes much more time, effort, and expenditure to attract a new customer, especially to draw one away from another organization, than it does to satisfy current customers.

Describing, or using marketing communications for attraction alone, could be counterproductive. If descriptions promise more than is delivered in the health care experience, dissatisfaction will likely result, with no lasting relationship. Moreover, dissatisfied customers probably will spread negative word-of-mouth advertising that will counter the health care organization's own marketing communications and reduce their effect on others. Given the effect of word-of-mouth communications on health care choices and behavior, it would be better to deliver without describing than to describe without delivering.

Relationship Marketing

In any service marketing situation, particularly when repeat and even regular service use is critical to the organization's success and survival, one can view marketing as *managing relationships.*[3] The purpose and types of relationships and whom they involve are functions of the organization's mission and conditions of its survival. The necessity and value of achieving and maintaining lasting relationships with identifiable groups motivate and justify the marketing effort.

All five marketing activities should serve relationship purposes:

- Discovering should focus on learning what publics want in a relationship, what it will take to get them to enter and remain in one, and how they feel about any existing relationship and about the health care organization doing the discovering.
- Deciding should determine with whom the health care organization wishes to build and maintain relationships, for what reasons, and on what bases.
- Designing should focus on developing and modifying what publics experience in their interactions with the organization in order to promote lasting relationships.
- Delivering should ensure that interactions are more than satisfy ing, so that publics will not look for new relationships.
- Describing should persuasively inform both prospects and current customers in ways that attract prospects and promote continuing relationships.

The Marketing Triangle

For hospitals, the essential customer marketing challenge requires managing a triangular relationship among the institution, physicians, and patients. Once this relationship was linear; physicians had patients and hospitals sought physicians who brought their patients with them. This is increasingly not the case as consumers assert themselves in making hospital choices and as hospitals can no longer rely on physicians having enough patients.

The effective marketing hospital must strive to create and maintain strong and lasting relations with its medical staff; this has not changed. It must also strive to create and maintain strong and lasting relations with patients and families, especially in high consumer choice services such as maternity. Moreover, the hospital should endeavor to promote strong and lasting relationships between its medical staff members and their patients, referrers, and other sources of business.

The triangle is the simplest and strongest basic structure in engineering. The hospital or other provider organization that can strengthen each side of the marketing triangle and manage the number and types of physicians, patients, and referrers can ensure its survival and mission achievement. The keys are knowing who has to be in the triangle and how to get and keep them in it.

The marketing triangle should probably be augmented to become a pyramid. The added dimension includes the health care organization's employees, nurses, technicians, and support personnel. Although in the truest sense they *are* the organization, it may be helpful to think of them as yet another focus of relationships. The organization's relationships with them can greatly influence how efficient, effective, and productive they are. It can also affect how they relate to patients and physicians, which in turn will affect how well the organization's relations with those two publics develop.

Similar logic applies to volunteers, donors, employers, and almost any other public who affects the health care organization. Marketing offers a set of principles; a way of thinking, acting, and communicating; and various techniques for managing relationships. The five basic Ds apply equally to all such relationships. The key is to plan and manage as many relationships as are necessary and effective in promoting the health care organization's mission and vitality.

Mission and Vitality

The religious health care organization, more than most other institutions, puts mission before survival, but it has to survive if its mission is to continue. When mission calls for serving the poor and powerless or any disadvantaged population underserved by other institutions, marketing can assist in attracting and satisfying:

1. Any special population the mission identifies or emphasizes.
2. Whatever other markets are required to promote survival in addition to mission.

If the organization is truly committed to serving the poor or any disadvantaged population, it can use marketing to promote its service. It is one thing to accept or even welcome patients that other providers avoid; deliberately cultivating such patients is something else. By consciously discovering what are the needs, wants, and wishes of a particular group, the organization can work toward increasing the probability that members of that group will seek needed health services and will come to that organization for them.

In many situations, the religious health care organization may find little competition, few if any other providers seeking to serve members of disadvantaged populations. Even where there are no competitors, members of the population may not be seeking all the care they need, or choosing the "right" provider. Deliberate marketing efforts aimed at such populations can increase the organization's success in carrying out its mission. Marketing to other populations may then be needed to improve the organization's likelihood of surviving.

The hospital truly committed to serving the needs of the poor can devote market research effort specifically to discover what services the poor desire, what characteristics of hospitals cause them to seek care rather than postpone or avoid it, and to prefer one hospital over another. The nursing home committed to caring for the needs of any disadvantaged population can devote its research, programming, and communications to attracting more of them. Meeting and exceeding the expectations of the poor will promote positive word-of-mouth advertising and help bring more of them to the organization's programs.

For greatest effectiveness in promoting both mission and survival, the organization must consider and understand each in terms of marketing dynamics. It must ask the following questions:

- How many of which group are to be attracted and satisfied in order to promote which aspects of mission or vitality?
- What has to be designed, delivered, and described to which persons in order to promote attraction and satisfaction?
- What unique or superior experiences can the health care organization offer so as to attract and satisfy enough of the intended markets?
- How can such experiences be delivered so as to promote vitality as well as mission?
- How can they be described in order to promote both attraction and satisfaction and to build lasting relationships?

The dual concerns of mission and survival further complicate the already complex challenge of marketing health care. Unlike most conventional marketing, health care has an extremely complex "customer," which can include patient, family members, physician, insurance company, employer, social agency, and government. Each customer component has slightly different and potentially conflicting needs, wants, and desires. Add to this the necessity of simultaneously focusing on mission and vitality rather than profit as a dominant motivation, and marketing health care is easily the most challenging of all marketing efforts. Many have long assumed that marketing came so late to health care because health care resisted; it may be that marketing looked at the situation and decided to try everywhere else first before tackling health care.

A Health Care Mission

The mission statements of many health care organizations are vague though admirable generalizations regarding the high purpose for which they were intended. Often they speak of "high-quality health care," "serving all who need health services," "addressing the full range of needs," or similar purposes. Such statements are important, but they do not go far enough. The mission, together with survival and vitality necessities, should form the basic motivation for all organizational decisions and activities. Topics at board and administrative meetings should reflect the institution's basic values, which should relate to either mission or vitality.

An organization's true mission is reflected in what it uses to evaluate its success and justify its decisions. If the minutes of meetings show that primary emphasis has been on financial considerations and that service decisions have been made based on where the greatest profit potential existed, then the organization's primary motivation may be prosperity or survival not service. If the organization evaluates and rewards employees and managers based on how productive and profitable their efforts have been, rather than on quality of care or service to the poor, then survival may have overshadowed or even replaced mission.

The mission should be a statement of commitments and obligations the organization has consciously embraced. At the same time, the organization should state the mission in terms that permit monitoring of success. A religious health care organization, committed to carrying out a healing ministry, should be able to check how well it is doing this year compared to last and should make decisions expected to result in doing better next year. To do so, the mission statement should cover who is to be served, what needs are to be addressed, and what services are to be offered. Vitality considerations and survival necessities may constrain how much of the mission the organization can accomplish and may even dictate that the service population and range of services be extended or limited. The mission statement should at least enable the organization to determine and report regularly how well it is achieving that mission, maintaining its vitality, and ensuring its survival.

Part of a religious health care organization's mission is likely at least to compromise its survival. Serving the poor or any population that promises less revenue than costs threatens the organization's vitality, at least in financial terms. Offering a range of services that includes some that are not self-supporting may do the same. Delivering a higher quality or fuller scope of service, such as including spiritual care, can also threaten survival, especially under fixed prospective payment systems, competitive bidding, or capitation payment arrangements.

The organization's mission should assist it in recruiting patients, employees, physicians, donors, and other sources of support who share its values. The more clearly the organization states such values, the more it promises, forecasts, and delivers accomplishments in such values, the more successful it should be in galvanizing support. One of the most important attraction features of a provider is a sense of trust and confidence in what it says and does. A religious health care organization should be able to generate a stronger sense of trust and confidence than most other institutions.

The religious health care organization, through its commitments to every individual's dignity and worth, may also labor under some handicaps in regard to its employee and physician relations. Commitments to employees' growth and development can be expensive. Concern for employees' families may interfere with maintaining minimum staffing levels during fluctuations in census. Commitments to equality of treatment may interfere with offering physicians attractive privileges that employees do not enjoy. Commitments to physicians' worth may motivate hospitals, for example, to rescue and restore an impaired physician, with attendant risk as well as potential benefit to the community and hospital.

On the other hand, commitments to dignity and worth may have distinct and significant benefits in terms of building strong and lasting relationships. Loyal employees and physicians can be more productive and contributive. They may engage in positive word-of-mouth advertising that strongly supports the organization's marketing efforts. They should help ensure that the care experience offered and delivered to patients is superior to that offered by institutions with poorer physician and employee relations.

Marketing is not a particularly moral discipline; it is a set of concepts, knowledge, and techniques that all kinds of people and organizations, both moral and immoral, can use. It can be and has been used for dubious purposes, for example, promoting the sale and use of alcohol and cigarettes, or worthless gadgets and baubles, including worthless cures and nostrums. It can and should be used for any high purpose as well. If marketing does offer any advantage to unethical or inferior health care providers, then it is all the more important that ethical and superior providers use it, and use it more effectively.

Attracting new patients, physicians, employees, and so on, is clearly vital to any provider's mission and vitality. Organizations can use marketing to attract more of any poor, underserved, or needy populations to services that will benefit them. Organizations can use marketing to attract sufficient volumes of patients to meet or surpass quality and efficiency standards and to promote financial achievements. Marketing can promote greater use of needed services by a given population, more appropriate use of services, or selection of more appropriate providers. It can help promote improved performance in the entire health care system, as well as in individual organizations.

Satisfaction is at least as valuable. Satisfied patients have better care outcomes, are less likely to sue, will use care more appropriately, will follow medical advice better, and will enjoy a higher quality of life than ones dissatisfied.[4] Satisfied patients, residents, and families promote continuity and thereby quality and efficiency of care and help in attracting more patients. Satisfied employees are more productive, efficient, and effective; satisfied physicians are more cooperative and loyal; and both enjoy their lives more.[5] Satisfaction is a necessary condition for the strong and lasting relationships essential to survival. In many instances, these relationships are equally essential to the organization's mission, or at least to optimum achievement of it.

Identification of the organization's essential values is basic to any marketing effort, just as it is basic to any planning and operational effort. Such values should include commitments derived from (1) the organization's sense of mission and purpose, (2) its understanding of the necessities of survival and vitality, and (3) its essential moral philosophy in regard to relations with persons and other organizations. The organization should be able to monitor all such values to determine its status at the beginning of any marketing effort and to evaluate how much progress it has achieved as a result of any such effort. This will probably be more difficult compared to monitoring only survival values and trusting good intentions to protect and further mission and moral values. Unless this monitoring is done, however, marketing may only help the organization survive and may pass up significant opportunities to help it succeed as well.

Footnotes

1. "AMA Board Approves New Marketing Definition." *Marketing News,* 19:5 March 1, 1985, p. 1.

2. Ries, A. and Trout, J. *Marketing Warfare.* New York: McGraw Hill Book Co., 1985.

3. Berry, L. "Relationship Marketing," in Berry, L. et al. (eds.) *Emerging Perspectives in Services Marketing.* Chicago: American Marketing Association, 1983, p. 25.

4. MacStravic, R.S. "Therapeutic Pampering." *Hospital & Health Services Administration* 33:3 (May/June 1986): 659.

5. Douma, A. "Informed Patients and Physician Satisfaction." *JAMA* 243:21 (June 6, 1980): 2168.

2. Discovering

Marketing focuses its attention on the organization's "customers," that is, the individuals and organizations whose behavior in the competitive marketplace determines how well the organization accomplishes its mission and whether it survives. The notion of customer can encompass financing and regulatory agencies, legislatures, foundations, and other organizations whose behavior affects the entire health care industry, in addition to employers, unions, banks, and so on whose behavior can affect individual institutions. Other customers include employees, hospital medical staff, donors, and volunteers who make up the organization. The major focus of marketing is attracting and satisfying persons in customer relationships; thus "customer" in this book includes all those who determine whether persons seek health care services and from which organization.

Even this limited definition of customer is based on the complex process and participants involved in health care choices. Patients, family members, personal physicians, employers, medical specialists, guardians, other institutions, and discharge planners may make or directly influence such choices. In addition, friends, co-workers, acquaintances and even strangers may supply advice or warnings that affect health care choices. Effective marketing must address as many of these participating and influencing persons as possible. Efficient marketing should focus on those persons it will have the most effect on for the least effort.

Leverage

Providers should concentrate their marketing efforts on the health care customers who promise the best results. The best "targets" of marketing efforts are those who (1) will most likely be attracted and satisfied and (2) will contribute most to mission success and survival if attracted and satisfied.

The physician's potential contribution is likely to be far greater than the average person. For example, one physician convinced that one hospital is the best place to admit patients may contribute hundreds of admissions per year. The average person has only a 10 percent chance of becoming an inpatient in any given year. Thus a physician may have a thousand times the leverage of an average citizen in terms of hospital use. Different physicians have different amounts of leverage. The active and successful internist, obstetrician, or general surgeon may contribute hundreds of admissions per year, whereas the dermatologist may contribute none or only a handful.

A discharge planner's contribution to a nursing home may be measured in dozens of residents referred per year, in hundreds of resident-days of care. Members of the clergy, gerontologists, social workers and other professionals working with the aged may have similar leverage. By contrast, the average citizen over age 65 has only about a five percent probability of being a nursing home patient. Attracting and satisfying a discharge planner, gerontologist, member of the clergy or social worker may have hundreds of times the leverage impact as persuading the average citizen.

Potential patients also differ in their leverage. For example, young persons are less likely to become inpatients than the elderly. Persons over 85 are far more likely to require nursing home care than those just over 65. For specific services, certain populations are significantly more at risk; that is, they have more leverage. Elderly people are more prone to seek ophthalmology services; middle-aged and older women, gynecology; younger women, obstetrics; young women, eating disorder care; and so on. Assuming it takes roughly the same effort to attract and satisfy any one individual, marketing should focus first on those who, once attracted and satisfied, will contribute the most to a health care organization's census.

In addition to leverage, there is the likelihood of attraction and satisfaction. For greatest marketing efficiency, providers should first seek those most likely to be attracted to and satisfied by what they offer and deliver. For example, current customers are more likely to contribute with less marketing effort than noncustomers. Attracting current patients to repeat use or additional services tends to be far easier and less costly than attracting new patients. Attracting new customers to existing services is probably easier than getting them to use new services, if they at least know of the organization's existing programs. Satisfying current patients is likely to be easier than satisfying new ones.

Thus a primary emphasis in all marketing effort should be on retaining existing customers. Attracting new ones may be essential, but so is keeping existing customers, and it probably will be much less expensive.

Attraction

The keys to attraction lie in two marketing concepts: the evoked set and the attribute set.

The *evoked set* is the collection of choices that come to the customer's mind under given circumstances, in some sequence or preference order. The focus of attraction efforts is on influencing which choices come to mind, under which circumstances, and in what order.

The *attribute set* is the collection of perceptions, both tangible and intangible, that cause persons to call to mind a particular set of options, to prefer one over others, and to determine whether they are satisfied with the choice. These perceptions may be accurate or inaccurate, rational reasons for preference or not, but they are significant enough to customers to affect their choices. As such, they are the logical targets of marketing actions and communications. To reinforce evoked sets that place one organization at the top, marketing may have to strengthen or change some actions and some messages. The key to effective and efficient marketing is to discover which actions and communications will do the most good.

Discovering Objectives

The discovering phase of marketing has four primary objectives:
1. Identify customers to discover who plays what role in determining how many of which group become guests of certain organizations for specific services
2. Learn what the evoked sets of such customers contain, under what circumstances they think of which service and provider options, and how they rank them
3. Discover which attributes determine provider preference and what perceptions customers have regarding competing providers
4. Learn what tangible features and sources of information most affect attribute perceptions

This section discusses these objectives in detail.

Customer Identification

Most organizations already have a good idea who their major (i.e., high-leverage) customers are. Providers tend to clearly identify and give special attention to repeat customers. The roles that guests, family members, and others play in making health care choices, however, may not be so well understood. Marketing offers, among others, two approaches to learning how customers make choices: focus group interviews and community or guest surveys.

Focus group interviews. These can be used with anyone participating in the health care decision. Although focus group experts describe many rules to follow, such groups are basically structured discussion groups.[1] A moderator chooses the structure and keeps the discussion focused on the intended topic. Participants may number from 6 to as many as 12 or more, depending on how many the group discussion can accommodate and involve. Rather than discuss in the abstract, the question of who plays what role in choosing providers, the moderator should use guests and their family members for the group. Discussion can then focus on how they chose the institution.

To avoid biasing the results, the group should include recent guests at competing organizations, and the discussion should take place at some neutral location, such as a hotel meeting room or other public place. Separate focus groups should be held to identify roles of different customers for different services; one group might consist of guests over age 65, whereas another might be recent maternity patients or surgery patients. The organization may use a different focus group for each product and market it serves. A focus group of physicians can give their insights into how they make service use and institution choices. These insights will probably be somewhat different from patients' perceptions.

Discussion questions for such focus groups might include the following:

- When it came time to select a (hospital, nursing home, other facility), who first suggested the one you chose?
- If the physician made the suggestion, did you bring up any other options? If so, what was the response?
- If the patient or family member made the suggestion, what was the physician's response?

The group discussion should trace how the guest selected the health care facility. The moderator should use chronological narrative and specific recall of conversations to reconstruct the process as thoroughly and accurately as possible. The results should provide insights into what roles different participants play in different situations. These situations include emergent ones, urgent and schedulable admissions, routine and life-threatening cases, admissions by family physicians and specialists, admissions from hospitals or family residences to nursing homes, or transfers from other homes.

Community or guest survey. The survey approach asks recent guests or a sample of community residents how they chose a recent hospital or other health service. The survey might offer specific options, such as:

- Choice was made by patient and family
- Choice was made by physician
- Choice was made jointly

If the respondent indicated a joint decision, the survey might probe further and ask: How would you describe how much the physician influenced the choice: only slightly, moderately, equally, more, or almost totally?

The organization should not treat such surveys as scientific proof but as indicators of relative influence on different types of choice situations. The purpose is only to help the organization decide where to place relative emphasis in marketing efforts.

Evoked Sets

Marketing may also employ both focus groups and surveys to identify evoked sets. The same groups and surveys may even be used for customer identification and evoked set identification. In both cases, the questions relate to what service and provider options persons call to mind under what circumstances and in what sequence or preference order.

The moderator might ask a maternity patient focus group to discuss: "When you consider(ed) where to deliver your baby, what options come (came) to mind?" To prevent one participant from biasing the group, each should write down her answers. The moderator should then ask participants to indicate which they think is the best choice or which one they chose. Similar questions can be used for other types of services and other guest or customer groups.

A survey can determine evoked sets in various ways. Any one or a combination of the following questions might be used:

- When you think of hospitals for (maternity care, surgical care, heart care, cancer care, child care, etc.), which ones come to mind?
- If a good friend asked you for the names of hospitals for (care category), which ones would you suggest?
- Which hospitals in the area offer (care category)?
- When you think of nursing homes, which ones come to mind?
- If a good friend asked you for the names of good nursing homes, which ones would you suggest?

Both the names of organizations mentioned and the order in which they are mentioned are useful information in evoked set identification. In most cases, the first one mentioned will turn out to be the one preferred, although exceptions occur.

To discover which organization people prefer, the survey can use different approaches:

- Which (hospital, nursing home) would you say is best?
- If you needed to be admitted (to a hospital for care category, to a nursing home), where would you go?

- If a good friend asked for your advice on where to go for (care category), which hospital would you recommend?

In most cases, the one preferred option will prove to be a significant factor in where people actually go for care, although the strength of preference may also be important. The survey can gauge strength by such questions as:

- If your physician recommended another institution, would you insist on your choice or follow that recommendation?
- If no beds were available at (preferred institution), would you go to another institution or wait until a bed became available?

All evoked set questions should be asked in the context of the specific circumstances under which the customer or guest makes specific service choices. If customer identification discoveries indicate that only physicians make neurosurgery, open heart surgery, or other highly specialized or life-threatening service choices, it makes little sense to ask for consumer preferences in such categories. On the other hand, evoked set questions are useful even for populations not at risk. For example, younger friends or acquaintances may ask women past childbearing age for advice. Thus, knowing and eventually influencing such persons' awareness and preference is still important, even if they are not prospective guests.

Attribute Sets

Discovering who significant customers are and what options they think of and prefer is a necessary beginning to a marketing effort. To influence preferences and behavior, however, it is essential to discover *what* produces preference. In most health care choices, when people think about their options, some combination of tangible and intangible attributes probably serves as the source of preference. *Tangible* attributes may include the institution's location, specific services offered, and whether one's personal physician is on the staff. *Intangible* perceptions or opinions are likely to include how reputable, competent, caring, comfortable, efficient, and reasonably priced, persons believe an institution to be.

Halo effect. A marketing effort must take into account what persons consider important and what they believe to be true about the provider. What is important to health professionals may not make a difference to guests; what is true may not coincide with what customers perceive. The discovering step should focus on learning what tangible and intangible attributes actually influence persons' preferences. In theory, this is a straightforward and logical step toward designing better patient care experiences and more effective marketing communications. In practice, it is enormously complicated by the *halo effect.*[2]

Some people might presume that persons arrive at their preferences by systematically considering the attributes of competing choices. In reality, this is not always true. Some may choose an institution entirely on the basis of another's recommendation, without developing a personal preference. Others may be taken to a hospital by ambulance, or they may ask a taxi driver to take them to the nearest one. When persons make choices before they have a preference, they tend to justify their choices by inventing preference and the perceptions that would justify such a preference after the fact. In any case, once people have an established preference, they tend to upgrade their positive perceptions of the preferred option and downgrade their perceptions of other choices.

This halo effect will be reflected in any focus group discussion or survey aimed at discovering why persons prefer one provider or service over others. At the time of the interview or survey, most persons have already established some notion of which is the best hospital. When asked what makes that hospital best, they are likely to mention attributes that justify and reinforce their preference, even though such attributes may have had little to do with how they came to prefer that hospital. Nursing homes are less well known by the public but probably have firm reputations among discharge planners, physicians, clergy, and others at the time any survey is conducted. Thus, in reality, discovery may be aimed at learning which tangible and intangible attributes *justify and reinforce* preferences rather than which ones caused them originally.

This aspect of discovery is not a futile exercise; it is essential to marketing. An institution can reinforce preferences of established customers and improve its rating among noncustomers only by discovering attributes people will report. Moreover, people are not likely to report irrelevant or insignificant attributes. Only the unconscious reasons for preference most likely will be missing from the discovery process. Since much is already known about unconscious motivation, marketers always can add that to what is discovered directly, although this introduces some interesting ethical questions, as discussed later in this chapter.

Marketers can ask various questions in focus group discussions or surveys to determine what attributes make the most difference to person's conscious preferences:

- What do you want most in a (hospital, nursing home)?
- What factors make (institution) the best choice?
- What made the most difference to your choice? (for recent guests and other customers)
- What one characteristic of (institution) makes it best?
- Are any other characteristics important as well?

If these questions are to be included in a focus group discussion, the moderator should request written answers before group discussion. Surveys should phrase such questions in an open-ended manner; otherwise, the language may bias the results.

Factors in provider preference. Based on hundreds of published studies and reinforced by my own market research efforts, most persons seem to give some fairly standard reasons for provider preference. They will vary in how they express these reasons, which are most important to them, and which they attribute to certain providers, but most reasons include:

1. *Competence factors*—qualifications, skill, experience in the particular service, facility offering that service
2. *Caring factors*—compassion, concern, friendliness, "being nice," attentiveness, responsiveness
3. *Convenience factors*—easy to reach, convenient hours, ease and safety of parking, short waits
4. *Continuity factors*—person always goes there, has personal physician on staff, knows personnel, is familiar with environment
5. *Cost factors*—reasonable and affordable charges, person's dignity and status not lost
6. *Comfort factors*—physical and psychological comfort (e.g., pain experienced vs. expected)
7. *Confidence factors*—reputable, effective, trustworthy, respected, popular institution
8. *Courtesy factors*—person feels respected, esteemed, important, worthy
9. *Control factors*—person given choice, allowed to participate in care and decision making
10. *Communicativeness factors*—person obtained desired information
11. *Commitment factors*—personnel interested, committed to identifying and responding to problems and needs

Customers will probably rate some factors as more important than others. Questioning can reveal the relative importance of factors in the attribute set, although unconscious motivators rarely emerge so easily. Such questions include:

- Which factors were most important in your choice?
- Of the factors mentioned, which was most important to you?
- Which was next? (etc.)

A useful approach in discovering important attributes is to record the order in which persons mentioned preference justification factors, without actually asking them to mention the most important first. This saves a step and may give a truer picture of what really influenced choice, rather than what persons might think should be most important.

The critical attributes that affect preference and choice are not necessarily the characteristics that are most important in an abstract sense, but those that distinguish competing providers in persons' minds. Most persons rate competence as most important, but this factor may not affect choice if all or many providers are viewed as roughly equal in competence. Marketing success depends on enough persons regarding the provider as significantly different or superior compared to other providers in some way, roughly equal in most areas, and inferior in no or only minor ways.

Satisfaction evaluation. Satisfaction should be addressed separately from attraction to some degree. Whereas efforts to discover what attracts customers focus on competing options, discovering their degree of satisfaction focuses on their recent experience. Marketers should use guest satisfaction surveys, on a systematic sample basis, to discover how satisfied guests and family members were with their institutional experience and which aspects most affected their feelings. Satisfaction of first-time and long-established customers is vital not only to their repeat use but to their word-of-mouth promotion of the institution.

Satisfaction monitoring should be systematic and continuous. Printed questionnaires can offer every patient and significant other (e.g., family, friend) a chance to comment on how they perceived a particular experience or feel about a continuing relationship. Sample phone or personal interviews can assess guest and other customer satisfaction in situations where sample numbers are sufficient to warrant confidence in results. If questionnaires are used, the marketer should instruct and motivate respondents so as to achieve close to 100 percent response. The typically low rate of return for most questionnaires carries with it a high risk of self-selection bias.

Satisfaction may be assessed on an overall basis only. For example, patients might be asked to indicate how they feel about their experience as a whole, with preprinted choices such as terrible, mostly dissatisfied, somewhat dissatisfied, mixed feelings, mostly satisfied, pleased, and delighted.[3] Such an approach tends to work better than asking persons to rate the organization or its personnel. Asking guests, family members, and other customers to report their feelings can elicit more subjective and accurate information.

If marketers want rating evaluations, they may employ a *scaled approach*. For example, patients might be asked: "On a scale of 1 to 10, where 1 means dreadful and 10 means wonderful, how would you rate your experience?" Another alternative is using an *agree-disagree approach*: "Please indicate whether you strongly agree, agree, have no opinion, disagree, or strongly disagree with the statement, "My experience as a patient (resident) was wonderful."

In addition to overall ratings, marketing may address specific judgment dimensions. Essentially the same dimensions as apply to attraction may be assessed in rating satisfaction, such as competence of personnel, caring, and comfort. Those dimensions deemed most important in attraction may not be equally important in satisfaction but should be assessed to provide information useful in managing word-of-mouth communications (see Chapter 6). From 2 or 3 up to 10 or 12 dimensions may be useful to assess, given persons' variability and what they value in guest and other customer experiences.

Whether an overall rating or specific dimension approach is used, all responses should be probed to identify the tangible factors that most influenced guest and other customer feelings. After each rating response, an interviewer might ask: "What one thing made the most difference to your (feeling, opinion, answer)?" Or "What was it about your experience that led you to rate it that way?" The marketer can try several different probing questions until one is found that consistently produces tangible and therefore actionable reasons for persons' intangible judgments. If questionnaires fail to produce such reasons, then phone or personal interviews should be used. Ratings alone are insufficient. Discovery should tell marketers what is helping and harming guest and other customer relations so they can act on the information.

Actionable and Communicable Features

Once it identifies customers and determines their evoked and attri-bute sets, discovery focuses on learning what objective, tangible, ac-tionable, and communicable features lie behind the attribute perceptions that explain the customers' preferences. Most preference-explaining perceptions tend to be intangible attributes, such as competence, caring, and convenience, expressed in judgmental and subjective terms: "The nurses really know what they were doing"; "People are nice"; "It's easy to get to." To decide, design, and deliver the most attractive and satisfying patient experience and to develop persuasive descriptions of it, market-ers must know what objective features cause people to reach which subjective judgments.

Marketers can identify tangible features that can be managed and communicated for marketing effect by interviewing either former patients or the public. Personal or focus group interviews may be effec-tive in boiling down subjective perceptions into objective features. Guest and family perceptions of nursing care may be traced to nurses answering call buttons promptly, giving back rubs, or knowing patients' names. Perceptions of physician competence may be traced to the physician's attentive listening, to the physician asking how the patient felt about the diagnosis or treatment, or to something as simple as the physician wearing a white coat.

In either focus interviews or surveys, questions should begin with a specific perception, then ask persons to report how they reached their conclusion regarding the factor involved. An interviewer might ask patients to rate the nursing staff on their competence or caring, then query "What did they say or do that caused you to rate them as you did?" After community residents rate the hospital or nursing home on com-petence or caring, the interviewer might ask: "How can you tell (institution) is (as rated)?" Gentle probing should be used until respondents shift from subjective, judgmental comments to objective, actionable items.

Information Sources

The final challenge in the discovery phase of attraction marketing is to learn what sources of information people use to develop perceptions of tangible and intangible attributes and to arrive at evoked set membership and order. Tracing established perceptions and preferences is not easy, since people's recollections of how they gained specific knowledge and attitudes are likely to be unreliable. To learn how people think they derived specific perceptions, an interviewer might ask the following:

- How did you learn that (institution) is (some tangible fact)?
- Have you or a member of your family ever been a patient/resident at (hospital/nursing home)?
- (If "no" answer to previous question) How did you determine that (hospital/nursing home) is (some intangible judgment)?
- What do you consider to be the most useful source of information about (hospitals/nursing homes)?

Based on published literature and my own patient and community research, the rank of information sources most people mention is as follows:

1. Personal experience as a patient or resident in the health care facility
2. Observed or vicarious experience as a family member or visitor
3. Specific advice or recommendation given by physician, other health or social service professional, family member, friend, or acquaintance on request
4. Unsolicited comments or general conversations about the institution participated in or overheard in the past
5. Newspaper, television, or other news or feature stories published in the local media
6. Direct mail advertising sent by the institution
7. Advertising in newspapers, television or other local media

Chapter 6 discusses information sources in more detail.

From these results, marketers should realize the importance of actual experience and word-of-mouth communications on persons' perceptions. Even when the volume and effectiveness of advertising and publicity efforts improve, persons probably will retain a high regard for their personal experiences and what they observed or heard from others. Most health care choices are sufficiently important that persons are unlikely to rely on advertising alone when making judgments. On the other hand, publicity may serve to influence word-of-mouth comments, to reinforce perceptions, or to supply relevant new information that may influence perceptions, preferences, and choices.

These information sources and their order of importance may not apply equally well to all categories of health care or to all providers. New programs and organizations are less likely to find personal or vicarious experience so important. For example, nursing homes are less likely to find that the public has had any prior experience with them, as compared to hospitals or medical practices. For these reasons, marketers should use questions on information sources in every discovery effort.

Unconscious Motivators

Thus far, the discovery step has concentrated on learning what conscious factors influence customer choice. Motivational researchers and behavioral scientists have clearly shown, however, that persons are motivated by a complex set of factors, the workings and impact of which they may not consciously perceive. Maslow's hierarchy of needs, for example, states that persons are motivated by needs for (1) physical well-being and survival, (2) safety and security, (3) love and belonging, (4) esteem by self and others, (5) self-actualization and achievement, and (6) knowledge and understanding and (7) aesthetic fulfillment.[4] People may not be consciously aware of how such needs influence their perceptions and preferences, but marketers must be aware of this.

For example, the most obvious motivators of choice are customers' perceptions of how they will be affected. In addition, however, persons are influenced by peer pressure—by perceptions about what others expect or wish them to do or about what is the popular choice.[5] Moreover, persons are influenced by symbolism, the meaning of alternate choices, and whether these choices fit with their self-image and contribute to their self-esteem.[6] Asking persons directly about peer preference and symbolism is unlikely to indicate the importance of these factors accurately, since these factors often work on a subconscious or unconscious level.

One way to gauge such factors' importance is to employ *forced-choice* interviews or surveys. The interviewer might ask customers to choose between two providers whose descriptions differed only in a single dimension. That dimension might be expressed in terms such as "has largest number of patients," "most popular," or "recommended by friends," to suggest peer preference. Symbolic meaning might be suggested by such descriptions as "has VIP suite," "recently used by popular TV star," or "the working person's/professional person's institution." If adding such a description to a list of otherwise identically or similarly described institutions produces a significant positive or negative impact on expressed choice, this suggests the impact of the peer preference or symbolism factor.

To gauge the relative importance of such factors compared to others, descriptions of competing providers would differ in two ways. One provider's description might contain a reflection of peer preference or symbolic meaning but lack a description of some other specific factor such as competence, caring, or convenience. The other provider's description would lack the peer preference or symbolic meaning suggestion but contain the other factor. By testing a series of forced choices and alternating the factors involved, the interviewer may obtain a suggestion as to the relative importance of such factors. This will only be a suggestion, since forced choices of hypothetical options involve oversimplified and artificial choices compared to actual customer preference situations.

The fact that peer preference and symbolic meaning impact on customer choices introduces some ethical questions. Using suggestions of such factors to market competing brands of beer, cigarettes, or perfume may not raise ethical issues, except for possible effects on overall consumption of harmful and useless products. In health care, however, substituting peer preference and symbolic meaning for essential factors that should influence customer choice runs counter to professional and organizational cultures. Since the factors are known to influence customer choice, two situations probably exist in which they may be appropriately used. First, if the organization has done its best to be excellent and be perceived as such on all other judgment dimensions, the peer preference and symbolism would be marketing frosting on an excellent cake. Second, if competitors are relying on peer preference or symbolism suggestions to market themselves, the organization may choose to counter such efforts with similar strategies.

It is an unfortunate but unavoidable reality that the organization that excels in objective measures of quality, convenience, caring, and so on must also excel in marketing if it is to enjoy the mission success and vitality it deserves. When peer preference and symbolic arguments can be added to rather than substituted for more "rational" bases for attracting and satisfying customers, no insurmountable barriers should arise. Each institution's values and traditions will provide the basis for making decisions regarding such use.

If the discovery effort is working well, the organization should learn much about how the market works, how customers make choices, and where it stands with current and potential customers. Moreover, such learning should be directly translatable into marketing decisions, design, delivery, and description strategies. To determine if this effort is effective, the organization should ask:
- Who are the logical target customers of our marketing efforts, given their leverage and likelihood of having their perceptions and preferences reinforced or altered? What effects on our mission and vitality will such reinforcement and alteration have?
- What do the evoked sets of such targets look like? Which organizations (e.g., hospitals, nursing homes) and service program options are listed, and in what order of recall and preference are they evoked?

- What do the attribute sets of such targets look like? Which tangible and intangible perceptions do they use in arriving at preferences? How do they perceive our organization compared to the other options in their evoked sets on intangible judgment dimensions?
- What tangible perceptions are responsible for target customers' intangible judgments about our organization and others?
- Which sources of information have influenced which perceptions? Which have had the greatest impact on preferences?

If the organization can confidently answer each of these questions, it will find that it is well prepared to carry out an effective and efficient marketing effort. This effort will focus on both guests and the customers who make and influence health care decisions and will be capable of enhancing both attraction and satisfaction. If the organization cannot answer these questions, it should allocate more time, effort, and resources to the discovery stage of marketing to prevent subsequent stages from being ineffective or overly expensive.

Discovery both begins and completes marketing efforts by supplying the information and understanding essential to the other four stages. It links specific marketing tactics to overall strategy and links the efforts aimed at one program or set of customers or guests to the organization's other efforts. It also serves the vital function of promoting individual and organizational learning, so that marketing efforts can become more effective and efficient over time.

Footnotes

1. Hisrich, R. and Peters, M. "Focus Groups: An Innovative Marketing Research Technique." *Hospital & Health Services Administration* 29:4 (July/Aug. 1982): 8.

2. Beckwith, N. and Lehman, D. "The Importance of Halo Effects in Multi-Attribute Attitude Models." *Journal of Marketing Research* 13 (Nov. 1976): 418.

3. Westbrook, R. "A Rating Scale for Measuring Product/Service Satisfaction." *Journal of Marketing* 44:3 (Fall 1980): 44.

4. Maslow, A. *Motivation and Personality* (2nd ed.). New York: Harper & Row, 1970, p. 38.

5. Ajzen, I. and Fishbein, M. *Understanding Attitudes and Predicting Social Behavior.* Englewood Cliffs, NJ: Prentice-Hall, 1980. p. 42.

6. Packard, V. *The Hidden Persuaders.* New York: Simon & Schuster, 1957.

3. Deciding

Strategic marketing is the primary deciding component of any marketing effort. It includes making basic decisions regarding the essential "business" of the organization, that is, its mission. It encompasses identifying necessities related to the organization's survival and maintaining its overall vitality. Finally, it involves specifying outcome objectives for the marketing effort and setting forth expectations about what marketing will accomplish. All three strategic decision challenges should be supported by systematic information inputs from the discovering component. Decisions then provide a structural foundation for the designing, delivering, and describing components to follow.

Mission Decisions

The most fundamental marketing decisions involve the organization's mission: its purpose for existing and continuing in operation. As noted earlier, religious health care organizations traditionally have admirable but rhetorical rather than practical mission statements. Such statements may refer to "healing ministries" or similar purposes that help unite the organization's managers and employees in a higher calling. From a marketing point of view, however, they may be sorely lacking in guidance for the critical questions related to (1) *who* are the organization's intended markets, (2) *what needs* it intends to serve, and (3) *what services* it intends to offer.

Mission statements should clarify the essential contributions that the organization is committed to making: the health of a population, the quality of life of specific groups, and the operation of the health care system. The mission should express the organization's fundamental values in terms of its service to others and should answer the questions: Who are those "others"? What service will be rendered to them? and What outcomes will the organization use to focus and evaluate its efforts? Mission statements may serve several legitimate purposes in addition to the guidance they offer to marketing. On the other hand, the extent and direction of guidance they offer to marketing efforts and to subsequent decisions on how the mission is to be carried out will have great impact on whether the mission is translated into action and whether the organization survives to continue its mission.

The "Who is to be served" question is a primary strategic marketing decision as well as a mission choice. The mission should specify the populations the institution intends to serve. Such populations may be described in terms of geopolitical units: as residents of identified towns, cities, counties, states, regions, or even countries. Service populations may also be described in terms of economic, demographic, or health status: the poor and powerless, the aged, children, expectant mothers, the terminally ill, or those suffering from diabetes, cancer, stroke, AIDS, or serious trauma. The institution may serve other groups in the natural course of operations, but would give the intended service populations special attention.

The population specified in the mission becomes the focus of systematic market analysis and success monitoring. Since they are the intended recipients of organizational services, marketing would insist on (1) systematic identification of their needs, (2) regular monitoring of the extent to which their needs are being adequately met, and (3) deliberate searching for opportunities to expand and improve service. In addition to the attention typically given to financial health, equal time should be given to reporting and discussing how well the organization is doing in its service mission. Marketing should focus as much on making sure the organization is serving its intended service population as on contributing to the organization's financial health.

Only by identifying the population to be served in systematic and specific language can marketing establish a *denominator* for identifying needs and monitoring mission achievements. Only by specifying the markets to be served can marketing examine needs for opportunities and discover effective bases for attracting and satisfying customers. As the system moves more toward denominator-based financing such as capitation systems, even the survival of the organization will depend on how well it serves an identified population.

Service Population

If the organization aspires to protecting and improving health, the service population is the denominator through which mortality, morbidity, and similar measures can be calculated. If the organization aspires to serving needs, the service population is the denominator whose needs it must address. If the organization desires a positive reputation, the service population represents those persons in whose minds this relevant reputation will have to be established and maintained. An organization can no longer ensure its survival merely by serving well all those who happen to be admitted for inpatient/resident care or show up for ambulatory services. For marketing and organizations to succeed, they must choose a specific population as the focus of marketing efforts and the basis for evaluating success.

In most cases, service populations should be broken down into significant categories based on differences in their needs or differences in organizational interest in them. If the mission places special emphasis on the poor, for example, then marketing should separate the poor from the rest of the population for analysis and marketing. Other *market segments* may be identified based on demographics (age, gender, place of residence, insurance or source of payment, etc.), health factors (disease, risk, needs, high vs. low use of health care, etc.), or psychographics (low vs. high interest in health, current loyal customers, those loyal to competitors, those without loyalty link, etc.). Each segment would then be examined, monitored, and addressed in different ways.

Needs Assessment

Two separate and complementary approaches are available for assessment of the mission or service population. The first is the traditional health professional approach, based on examining health status, from physical and emotional to social and spiritual components. Experts identify such needs through vital statistics, systematic health examinations, quality of life indexes, and so on. A *need* in such a context is defined as *a discrepancy between a person's or a population's actual status on some objective measure and what the system believes this status can and should be.* Traditional community health planning formerly focused on this definition of need before it shifted to a regulatory mission focused on limiting health care resources.

The second approach to needs assessment comes from marketing and focuses on the self-defined needs of the mission population. Such needs may be for specific services, such as wellness, cosmetic, or other services enhancing the quality of life, that go beyond what health professionals would characterize as needs. They are also likely to include needs that arise from persons' perceptions of and attitudes toward how professionally defined health needs are being met. From a marketing perspective, a person dissatisfied with a current system of health care or provider "needs" a better choice.

The professional approach to needs assessment is designed to identify potential obligations the organization might take on. The institution would assess its potential for successfully addressing a given health need, improving health status, preventing disease or damage, or at least minimizing the effects of conditions that can neither be prevented nor cured. The marketing approach is designed to identify potential opportunities the organization might pursue. The institution would assess whether it can do better than it or its colleagues are currently doing and what this could contribute to its mission and survival.

Mission Needs and Services

Needs to be addressed and services to be offered further define mission, once it has identified the populations with needs who can use services. Organizations may consciously expand or contract the range of needs they intend to address, and the scope of services they intend to offer. The organization should base decisions in both areas on its mission, on needs assessment discoveries, and on practical considerations related to the foreseeable impact of needs/services decisions on its vitality.

The Traditional Hospital Today

In its traditional form, the hospital has only one characteristic that makes it unique in the health care system: the provision of 24-hour acute nursing care. It also has, in most cases, a role that makes it at least unusual: 24-hour medical care. The hospital is facing increasing competitive pressures in almost every other service area as freestanding "boutiques" specializing in selective populations and services spring up on every corner. The 24-hour franchises that hospitals retain are unlikely to be sufficient, either to their mission or to their future survival, under the combined onslaughts of reduced willingness to pay and increased competition. A mission to address the health needs of an identified population systematically and comprehensively should present an enormous array of potential obligations and opportunities. The organization is challenged to select and assert its role in meeting that population's total health needs. It should enjoy some competitive advantages in doing so: established tradition; good reputation; positive relations with physicians, patients, and community; closely related services; one-stop convenience for multiple needs; and so on. It is also likely to suffer from some significant disadvantages: high costs, inexperience or uncertainty in competitive marketing, and dependence on medical staff members who may also be fierce competitors.

The hospital has the potential for exploiting its franchise advantages and living within the constraints of its competitive disadvantages. As the sole source of 24-hour acute nursing care and whatever high-technology services it monopolizes, the hospital is likely to be the only possible source of truly comprehensive health care for any given population. As such, it is uniquely capable of becoming the fulcrum for a comprehensive, integrated delivery system, offering personal and family continuity in contrast to the single-focus, fragmented nonsystem that boutiques represent.[1]

The hospital need not and should not attempt to provide all services in a comprehensive system. Because it relies on medical staff and because it is simply not the best place to deliver all services, the hospital should network with other providers, including selected boutiques, as appropriate. As the payment system moves toward capitation/ competitive bidding, the most effectively and efficiently integrated system is the one that will achieve the greatest marketing success and highest probability of survival.

The Traditional Nursing Home Today

Nursing homes, like hospitals, are seeing their competitive positions eroded even as an aging population and DRG payment systems for hospital inpatient care stimulate potential demand for their services. Because of the high costs of nursing home care, and given the frequent scandals or questionable reputations involving some homes, alternative forms of care are being promoted by practically everybody. As certificate-of-need laws and programs disappear, new nursing homes are springing up where before the supply was kept to a minimum. Hospitals are converting their unused acute care beds to long term care.

The traditional nursing home neither needed nor invested in much marketing effort. In the future, homes will be forced to expend far greater effort toward attracting and satisfying their customers. They should investigate offering home health care, respite and day care, and ambulatory services in addition to conventional resident care. They can work toward developing or becoming parts of vertically integrated systems oriented toward the needs of the elderly population in general, including assisted living, retirement, and life care communities.

Choosing Services

The traditionally recommended approach to making hard-headed business decisions regarding which services to offer is the technique of *portfolio analysis*.[2] This technique examines each identifiable *strategic business unit* (SBU) or product line of the hospital as a separate business investment. It fails in at least two ways, however, as an adequate basis for needs and services decisions in health care. First, portfolio analysis fails to consider the medical and marketing interdependencies among specific services. Second, it fails to ask why any given service, at the time it is examined, is low in market share, growth, or profitability; thus it does not address whether a potential exists for changing rather than accepting the situation and its implications.

The interdependence of separate services is perhaps best illustrated by maternity care programs. Maternity has traditionally been a low-profit or even loss-leader service in most hospitals. As a market, it has been in a state of decline for a long time as family size has decreased and average length of stay has declined. Moreover, competition from freestanding birthing centers and home deliveries has cut into that declining market. Also, conventional wisdom has long asserted that fewer providers of maternity care with higher volume per provider is the best way to ensure high quality. Thus many hospitals have dropped their obstetric programs for survival or public service reasons.

From a marketing perspective, the lack of obstetrics is a serious disadvantage. First, it precludes the hospital from being a "full-service" institution. Second, it tends to produce an accompanying decline in pediatrics and gynecology. Third, and perhaps most important, it deprives the hospital of the best possible opportunity to initiate a lasting relationship with its mission population, unless that population includes no potential parents. The experience of childbirth, with its long lead time and opportunities for parenting and childbirth classes and its usually happy outcomes and family involvement, presents an excellent opportunity for the institution to become the mother's, father's, child's, and even other relatives' favorite hospital. Without such an opportunity, a hospital is forced to overcome the lead of its competitors.

The hospital may have to adopt the type of programs mothers want, including same-room labor-delivery-recovery suites, short-stay maternity options, and others in order to compete with freestanding alternatives. The hospital should organize and operate maternity programs as fundamental components in its marketing strategy of becoming the personal hospital of as many persons in its mission population as possible. Unless financial losses make continued operation impossible, the hospital should be adamant in refusing to give maternity services up. The volume-quality linkages that have promoted the closure of obstetric units in the United States are highly questionable, given studies in other countries and the experience of freestanding centers that often operate with lower volumes than hospitals had before they closed their units.

A similar logic applies to hospital emergency rooms (ERs). As freestanding urgicenters and minor emergency/convenience clinics have proliferated and private physicians have responded by extending their hours and offering walk-in appointments, the ER as a medical convenience center has suffered market losses. At the same time, the quality of care advantages of having 24-hour medical coverage for inpatients, and the marketing advantages of being open to ambulances and emergency patients at any hour make an ER a service that should not be discontinued without intensive consideration. The indirect effects on community trust in the hospital, on inpatient admissions, and on coverage of current inpatients may be far more negative than any financial losses saved by closing the ER.

Implications of Service/Need Decisions

Any service/need decision will affect both the mission and the survival of the organization. The full effects of any such decision on marketing, as well as on operations, strategic ambitions toward becoming a comprehensive and integrated delivery system, and immediate financial health, should be identified and evaluated. Moreover, the organization should scrutinize the reasons for any disappointing program statistics. Financial losses in maternity or emergency programs may be reversible through better management, more effective marketing, or both. Even a declining or stagnant market may be stimulated through community education and marketing communications. It may be easier to make service/need decisions on the basis of current profitability and contributions without considering side effects or change potential, but it is irresponsible and dangerous to do so.

It is also irresponsible and dangerous for organizations to make service/need decisions without considering their survival and the mission implications. The mission may call for the organization to offer specific services or address specific needs. If beginning or continuing to offer such services and address such needs threatens the organization's vitality and future and its ability to continue its mission, it would be poor strategy to allow short-term mission commitments to dictate decisions. In pursuit of a position as sponsor, leader, or even participant in a comprehensive and integrated provider system, the organization can comfortably decide not to be the provider of individual services, as long as the system is doing so in an acceptable and viable manner.

Even decisions regarding who belongs in the mission population and what mix of patients are to be served should be made in light of survival as well as mission requirements. To serve the poor and those with limited ability to pay, the institution must also serve enough of those with full or at least greater ability to pay. When the individual institution reaches the limits of its ability to subsidize charity care, it may have to rely on a system approach, just as is the case with individual service/need decisions. Lobbying for legislation, community fund raising, and networking with other providers should supplement the organization's own charity care wherever needed and appropriate.

Mission decisions should never be considered as immutable; both circumstances and the organization's survival may make change essential and appropriate. The underlying values of the organization may remain constant; however, the organization should regularly reconsider specific decisions regarding who belongs in the mission population, and how many needs are addressed through which services, and which services belong in the mission statement. Missions are fulfilled when needs are met and services are rendered, even if by other providers. Survival necessities as well as mission aspirations require marketing logic and effectiveness as well as goodwill.

Strategic Goals and Objectives

Conventional wisdom in strategic planning insists that all goals and objectives be quantified. Thus marketing should consider only goals and objectives capable of quantification and, when formulated, should state them in specific, measurable terms. For example, increasing market shares is not enough; it is vital to increase them from some *percentage* to a higher percentage. This notion can be overstated, however, and force strategy into an artificial and arbitrary mode. The only requirement is that strategies should always aim at measurable value outcomes.

The values of organizations should be expressed in mission and service/need decisions and, even more importantly, in strategic goals and objectives. The mission statement may express what the organization would like its mission to be; it may cite philosophical values that unite its members in common cause and make them feel good about continuing and enhancing its operation. Service/need decisions and particularly the organization's strategic goals and objectives determine what the mission actually accomplishes. The organization's true mission is what it spends its energies and resources on, what it monitors systematically, and what it sets goals and objectives for.

Strategic goals and objectives should address both mission and vitality values. The organization should identify each value in measurable terms, identify the current status of each, and decide which ones it wants to improve. Such improvement may take two forms: making it better or keeping it from getting worse. Both require developing as clear a notion as possible regarding the expected future status of each value without intervention, a "business-as-usual" forecast. The goals and objectives are (1) value states that are better than what would occur if present activities were maintained and (2) the bases for determining how much change in current activities is necessary and worthwhile.

Mission Goals and Objectives

If their missions differ, it is inevitable that organizations' goals and objectives differ. Most mission goals and objectives will include aspirations regarding one or more of the following values:

- *Contributions to health:* external measures of outcomes such as mortality, morbidity, health status, and life quality improvements in the mission population attributable to the organization's programs

- *Quality:* internal measures of excellence in resources (medical staff, employees, facilities, equipment), process (protocols established and followed), and outcomes (infection rates, morbidity, mortality, complications, home discharges)
- *Status:* leadership, dominance, and respect in the community and among peers
- *Relationships:* with medical staff, employees, volunteers, auxiliaries, donors, employers, community leaders, and other provider organizations
- *Service:* categories of service offered, extent of use, share of markets per product line, and percentage of mission population's needs addressed

In any organization at any time, some of the "values," those goals worth pursuing and maintaining, may be considered either mission or survival values. The difference is entirely in how organizations regard them. Any value worth pursuing in and of itself, an *intrinsic value,* is a mission value. If everyone understands why the organization is pursuing a value, and it clearly should be continually pursued toward some ultimate perfection, then the value is an intrinsic, mission value. If why an organization pursues something relates to achieving a better status of that thing to produce some other worthy outcome, then that thing is an *instrumental value.* This value presumably is related to the organization's survival and vitality.

Status, for example, may be valued and pursued in its own right or as a way of ensuring continued operation. Relations with guests, medical staff members, or employees, may be valued in their own right or purely as a way to enhance use and productivity. The organization may develop and market services and identify and serve populations only to generate revenues to maintain other services or to subsidize services to other populations. In many cases, the distinction between intrinsic and instrumental values is unclear. This should present no problem in practice until values come into conflict or competition, when distinguishing one from the other can be helpful.

In most cases, the distinction between intrinsic, mission values and instrumental, vitality values will be clarified by how far the institution pursues them. In any religious or even community not-for-profit organization, financial values should be instrumental and pursued only up to some level necessary and appropriate to organizational vitality. For-profit organizations might have goals calling for net profits to increase by 20 percent per year. This strongly indicates that profit is an intrinsic value and essential part of their mission. The religious health care organization is more likely to set a goal calling for net revenues of some amount or percentage of revenues and work to achieve and maintain that level, but not surpass it. An instrumental value is pursued until enough has been achieved; maintenance then follows. An intrinsic value is pursued until no more improvement is possible or realistic; it serves as a constant source of motivation.

Vitality Goals and Objectives

An organization at a given time might identify almost any of the previously cited mission goal and objective values as vitality goals. In addition, most organizations will probably formulate vitality goals and objectives in the following categories:

- *Financial:* access to capital, reserves, profitability, cash flow/ liquidity, debt/equity measures, and similar reflections of financial health
- *Utilization:* internal measures of marketing effect, as determined by admissions, length of stay, ambulatory visits, surgeries, diagnostic and therapeutic procedures, and so on
- *Productivity/efficiency:* traditional operational measures directly affected by marketing success, such as occupancy level, since volume of utilization largely determines the efficiency of any operation
- *Satisfaction/morale:* attitudes of guests, medical staff, volunteers, and other personnel (Even if not valued in their own right, these are vital to marketing and management success.)

Although many of these vitality values have traditionally been used as reflections of management performance, they are equally functions of marketing. Financial health is as much determined by how many and what kinds of guests, physicians, employees, and others have been attracted and satisfied as by how well organizational management controls income and expenditures. Utilization is initially a function of marketing success in attracting and satisfying customers, although it may also be a function of case management efforts by hospitals and physicians in the interest of containing cost. Productivity is limited to the volumes that marketing brings in, whereas satisfaction is the particular focus of marketing efforts, whether under the rubrics of guest, professional, or employee relations.

In strategic marketing, decisions focus on the mission and vitality values that the marketing effort protects or enhances. One or more of such values should serve as the initial motivation and focus for marketing efforts. If this is the case, the marketer may formulate a quantified objective (but in pencil or erasable ink). In the long run, the outcomes or mission and vitality objectives achieved through marketing effort must be worth the cost of such effort. Thus it is reasonable to avoid specifying a quantitative objective at the beginning of formulating a marketing strategy and program. Instead, it may work as well to specify how much of an outcome is needed to justify the expense of whatever strategy and program is developed, once its costs have been estimated.

Marketing Objectives

Mission and vitality objectives must be translated into marketing terms as a basis for formulating marketing strategies. For example, the marketer might first translate a contribution objective related to improved health status into a utilization objective involving participation in an education or prevention program, or visits to a diagnostic or treatment program. A financial objective might be translated into a utilization (or perhaps a donation) objective. The marketer would then translate these into marketing objectives, specifying how many persons in a given market should register in or be admitted to a given program or seek care at the organization. This produces the utilization outcome that will yield the contribution or financial outcome desired.

A marketing objective is a statement of a pattern of market choices made by members of an intended mission population or customer group. It should reflect the total potential choices, enabling a calculation of the share of market needed to achieve the marketing objective. If an inpatient program requires 1,000 admissions, for example, in order to produce some desired quality, efficiency, revenue, or contribution to health outcome, then the marketing objective is to attract 1,000 admissions. If a total of 10,000 such admissions are expected in the market served by the hospital, then the marketing objective translates into a share of 10 percent. Both the number of market decisions required and the share of all expected decisions provide the focus for developing marketing design, delivery, and description strategies.

Any mission or vitality objective that can be achieved or approached through marketing can be translated into a pattern of market choices needed out of the total choices made. Marketing may accomplish a given objective through any combination of influencing the total number of such choices (*market strategies*) and the pattern of provider selection (*share strategies*). For example, a diabetes control program may grow by increasing screening and education that identifies more of the estimated 5 million undiscovered cases of type II diabetes. A provider that merely hangs on to its present share of the diabetes market can expect increased utilization when the market increases. For acute inpatient programs, however, the focus must be on maintaining or increasing share in a stagnant or declining market, despite increased competition. In contrast, nursing homes enjoy an increasing market population, despite increasing competition from noninstitutional providers and the government's growing reluctance to pay for nursing home care.

Attraction and Satisfaction Objectives

Each marketing objective should be translatable into some combination of attraction and satisfaction objectives. To maintain volumes of utilization attributable to established customers, the institution must satisfy those customers enough to ensure they will not go elsewhere. To achieve volumes of utilization attributable to new customers, the institution must attract such prospective customers enough to ensure they will prefer the organization to their other options.

Evoked Set Positions

Attraction and satisfaction states exist in the minds of the customers involved in making market choices. In health care this includes patients, payers, physicians, family, and professional advisers, who have varying influence in any one market decision and varying involvement in such decisions—that is, varying leverage. If an average of three persons are involved in a given health care market decision, then three attraction and satisfaction challenges exist per decision. One may view these challenges as achieving one of five evoked set positions that the organization or its programs may aspire to in the minds of customers who participate in specific health care choices:

1. Only known option
2. Top-of-mind option
3. Acceptable option
4. Best option
5. Only acceptable option

1. These positions are listed in ascending order of difficulty and value to the organization. Becoming the *only known option* to some segment of a market or group of choice participants requires little more than marketing communications. A sufficient volume of publicity, advertising, personal selling, and word-of-mouth communications can make a provider the only source of a particular service known by a particular group. This is greatly assisted if the provider *is* the only available source, at least in the immediate vicinity, and if customers make choices without considering much more than availability. It also requires that any other sources of the same service keep quiet about it, thereby not becoming known as another option and cluttering up customers' evoked sets. Such cooperation is rare, unless competing providers lack interest in attracting new customers and guests.

Being the only known source of care to some significant market segment can produce substantial marketing success by itself. For certain routine types of care, or wherever persons lack time, inclination, or both to seek out other options, being the sole occupant of an evoked set should lead to getting the business. One study, for example, indicated that 78 percent of families choosing a nursing home considered only one home.[3] If choices based on sole known source are not fully satisfactory to guests or other customers, however, this may stimulate searches for other sources. Moreover, if any competitor's market research identifies a substantial group who know of only one outside option, the competitor will almost surely decide to undertake the effort needed to become another known option. If two or more options are present in people's evoked sets, it is useful to at least achieve a top-of-mind position.

2. The *top-of-mind position* is similar to that of only known option in that it is based on knowledge alone, with no feelings, attitudes, or preferences involved. Top-of-mind merely means the first option that comes to mind and can be based on name recognition, familiarity, or reputation alone. It is a competitive position in that it requires being better known and more familiar than other known options. Top-of-mind position may be based on being more clearly associated with the decision maker's particular need or service, or even being known as the more comprehensive or full-service provider and therefore more likely to be able to address a given need. It is effective only if customers turn to the top-of-mind choice without carefully considering alternatives to reach a reasoned preference.

Top-of-mind positions based on familiarity alone are likely to be short-lived in any competitive situation. The providers who fall below the top position in familiarity are likely to seek that position through aggressive marketing communications or to suggest reasons for customers to prefer them to the most familiar option. Whenever customers have the time, motivation, and information to arrive at a preference among competing options, being the first to come to mind will not be enough.

3. Being viewed at least as an *acceptable option* means that the decision maker is aware of two or more possibilities and has screened them to eliminate any clearly unacceptable options. The person may view those that pass the screening process as roughly equivalent on all important choice dimensions. If so, a single factor such as convenience of location, being first in the alphabet, or almost any trivial factor may lead to the choice. The key to being in the set of acceptable choices is to avoid being linked to any negative perceptions. A nursing home or physician, for example, may be chosen when others are busy and require an extended wait. If customers are going to rank the options that are acceptable, the provider should strive to be the best or only appropriate option.

4. Being considered the *best option* is the aim in any marketing challenge involving persons who consider their options carefully before acting. When sheer volume of communication suffices to establish only known or top-of-mind positions, being the best choice means the provider must make deciders justify to themselves why they ranked the provider first among carefully considered options. Usually this requires becoming known for at least one significant distinction, such as offering a unique service or superior feature.

Being the top-ranked choice in persons' evoked sets usually indicates a high probability of getting the business when the need for care occurs. If another option is viewed as almost as good or barriers to use of the preferred option occur, (e.g., all beds are full, a two-week wait for an appointment), the second-ranked option may be chosen instead. If a provider is best but is not far above another choice, the provider should work on eliminating barriers to use in order to achieve the most out of a customer's mild preference.

5. A position as the *only acceptable option* involves such a strong preference that persons would not use other options even if barriers to the preferred option existed. Persons may base this decision on perceptions that give the preferred choice substantial distinctions and superiorities in major judgment dimensions. Persons may also have significant negative perceptions regarding other options, in which case one is not so much preferred as others are rejected. In most cases, anyone who regards a provider as the only acceptable option will choose that provider. Such a strong preference in the mind of even one participant involved in a group choice may sway other participants. Given the many participants in most health care decisions, however, it is unsafe to rely on achieving such a position in the mind of only one.

Being viewed as the only acceptable choice is likely to be a longer-lasting and more effective position in people's evoked sets. The competitor wishing to displace the provider in such a position would have to offer something dramatically new in the way of information, argument, or service. If the number one choice lapses into arrogance or complacency, however, the competitor's task is greatly simplified.

Unfortunately in health care, achieving the desired position in someone's mind does not necessarily translate into use of services. A potential nursing home resident may prefer one institution but be forced to go elsewhere because of financial reasons, lack of available beds, or family pressures. A potential patient may prefer one hospital but go to another because of an emergency, specific service needs, physician advice, or other reasons. Marketing effort can succeed in making one provider the one preferred by potential guests and customers, but it may not be able to control the circumstances that ultimately determine where they go for care.

Deciding from Position Characteristics

The discovering phase of marketing should identify which position the provider occupies in the minds of which decision participants. It should also identify the specific perceptions of distinctions or superiority that account for any preference discovered. Finally, discovering should identify, or at least suggest, what tangible characteristics of preferred and nonpreferred options make the most difference to perceptions and preference ranking. Given such information, the decision phase can then determine the markets most likely to be satisfied and retained and most likely to be attracted.

Attraction marketing efforts should focus first on higher-leverage customers who (1) are dissatisfied with their present options, (2) know of only one option that happens to be a competitor, (3) place a competitor at the top of their minds without preference, or (4) have only a mild preference toward a competitor, in that order. If the only available markets have a strong or overwhelming preference for competitors, it will take far more dramatic effort to attract them away and far less competitive response to prevent it. The cost of marketing effort compared to the expected impact, given probable competitive responses, is likely to represent a dubious bargain under such circumstances.

Satisfaction efforts should focus on reinforcing high levels of satisfaction if they are based on what is presently delivered. Also, a provider should be able to sway slightly dissatisfied customers easily and inexpensively, thus moving as many people as possible from considering the provider their best choice to rating it the only acceptable choice. By strengthening satisfaction, such efforts will in turn support attraction efforts by promoting positive word-of-mouth communications.

Strategy Selection

A marketing strategy includes identification of the market to be pursued or retained and specification of the basic approach to be used in doing so. Strategies for new services may rely on communications alone, achieving attraction as the only known option, then focus on achieving high levels of satisfaction to make it difficult for competitors to enter the same market. Strategies for services with high degrees of only known and top-of-mind positions may focus on out-communicating the competition or on developing and becoming known for some significant distinction or superiority.

To overcome preference of competing options, organizations should select one or more intangible judgment dimensions or tangible features on which they can develop and maintain a significant distinction or superiority. Any one of the dimensions listed in Chapter 2 may serve. Tangible features such as charges, hours, scope of services, and locations, may directly affect preference, influence intangible judgments, or both. Thus a strategy may be named after an intangible dimension, such as a convenience, caring, competence, or comfort strategy. It might also be named after the tangible feature that serves as a focus: a locations strategy, an extended-hours strategy, a comprehensiveness or pricing strategy, and so on.

If more than one market segment or participant group is the focus of a marketing effort, the provider probably will need more than one marketing strategy. Different segments and customers most likely have different values and expectations and require different tangible and intangible distinctions and superiorities to change their minds. Thus an effort united by a single marketing objective may require several separate marketing strategies. All should focus on the same objective but address the segments and customer groups who must alter their evoked and attribute sets if the objective is to be achieved.

The deciding phase, if properly executed and based on quality information inputs from the discovering phase, should set the tone and provide the framework for the designing and delivering phases to follow. A competence strategy, for example, would require designing and delivering features that will communicate competence to the intended markets. A price strategy would have to design and deliver features that would reduce prices to the market without undermining revenue to the provider. The design phase translates strategic decisions into program features that can be delivered with intended marketing effect at acceptable management cost.

A nursing home may aim to become the center of an ongoing system of support services to the frail elderly population in its service area. Using the institution as a base, it may develop or network with programs, including home care, durable medical equipment (DME) rental and sales, congregate care, hospice services, respite care, and activities programs. Such programs may generate additional revenue and may even be profitable in their own right, in addition to making the institution well known and liked in the area.

Footnotes

1. "Vertically Integrated Delivery System." *Healthcare Marketing Report* 2:12 (Dec. 1984): 1.

2. MacStravic, R.S., Mahn, E. and Reedal, D. "Portfolio Analysis for Hospitals." *Health Care Management Review* (Fall 1983): 67.

3. Froebe, D. et al. "Variables Influencing the Consumer's Choice of Nursing Homes." *Journal of Health Care Marketing* 2:2 (Spring 1982): 25.

4.Designing

The discovery phase of marketing should have answered the following:

1. Who in the market has what influence on which health care decisions?
2. Where are the provider and its programs positioned in the minds of which segments (only known, top-of-mind, acceptable alternative, best, or only acceptable option)?
3. What specific tangible features and intangible judgments had what effect on the provider's preference position?

The decision phase should have used these answers, together with explicit notions of the organization's mission and vitality, to answer:

1. What mission and vitality values ought to be protected or enhanced and to what degree through markering effort?
2. How many of which people should be targeted for marketing effort to achieve mission and vitality objectives?
3. Should such effort be aimed at attraction or satisfaction preference positions?
4. What basic areas of distinction or superiority will be the focus of marketing effort?

Once these two phases are completed (in draft and pencil so that changes can be made easily on the basis of subsequent choices), the design phase is responsible for choosing the specific program and institutional actions that will be taken. The purpose and focus of such action is to provide the basis for becoming or remaining the best or only acceptable choice in the minds of the selected strategic targets. If positions as the only known or top-of-mind option are desired, marketing communications alone may suffice, so marketing effort could skip to the description phase.

Tangibles and Intangibles

Providers can choose from three basic categories of actions to design the kinds of guest or other customer experiences that will help achieve marketing objectives:

1. The most straightforward category involves actions directed at specific tangible perceptions: better products, place, or price experiences in objective terms.
2. Actions aimed at specific semitangible perceptions, in which the focus of actions is clear but patient and other customer judgment is uncertain.
3. Actions directed at intangible judgments where the connection between tangible features and intangible judgments is likely to be diffuse and unpredictable.

Tangible Features for Tangible Perception Effects

The easiest areas for marketing design involve tangible provider and program features, the importance and preference effects of which can be directly measured. Marketing can employ several research techniques to identify the tangible features that make the most difference to marketing targets, including the focus group interviews and customer surveys described in Chapter 2. In addition, a handful of quantitative techniques can identify what levels and mix of tangible features are most attractive and satisfying to specific segments. This determines what levels of features make what difference to overall preference.

Marketing has used conjoint, functional, and LOGIT analysis in specific health care design situations to discover insights on how specific tangible aspects of a health care experience will affect preferences.[1] The mechanics of the analysis are beyond the scope of this book but can be handled by any sophisticated computer analyst familiar with marketing research techniques. The mechanics of collecting the necessary data inputs, however, are fairly simple.

The first step is to identify a set of tangible features which may take one of at least two alternative discrete forms (e.g., provider is a physician or a nurse practitioner) or a variety of continuous forms (e.g., charges of $25, $35, $45 per visit). The results of focus group discussions or customer surveys should produce suggestions for the types of features and discrete or continuous forms to which decision makers are sensitive. The provider then must determine what range of options it wishes to ask about, based on what is feasible and consistent with its mission and vitality values.

To illustrate, in designing a maternity experience for marketing to expectant mothers, the most critical tangible features might be location of the hospital or birthing center, choice of birthing experiences, charges, and providers. Within each feature category, three representative options may exist:

Location—5, 10, or 20 minutes away

Experiences—traditional, natural, and homelike

Charges—$1500, $2000, $2500 packages

Providers—obstetrician, family practitioner, nurse midwife

With three levels on each of four features, a total of $3^4 = 81$ possible mixes of program options would be available for preference rating. If the number of features or levels were greater, even more possibilities would be available.

Fortunately, there are ways to reduce the number of possible options to a manageable number, usually around 30. Both an *orthogonal array* and a *fractional factorial design* may be used to achieve this reduction. Again, a market researcher familiar with these techniques should be able to help in developing the selection set. The representative set of program choices is given to samples of prospective and present customers. Members of this sample then organize the option in priority order (*conjoint*) or rate them on some assigned interval or ratio scale (*functional*). The rankings or ratings of the entire sample are then analyzed by computer (the MONANOVA algorithm is typically used.)

If persons tend to rate or rank highly all options that are located nearby before they begin discriminating among options that are of different prices, for example, they are displaying a higher sensitivity to location than to price. If all options 20 minutes away are rated at the bottom, regardless of their other features, then location would be considered the most dominant feature. The quantitative analysis techniques discover patterns in the ratings or rankings of diverse options that reveal the underlying importance of specific features, even if persons may be unconscious of how such features affect them. In this way, the results of such analyses may be more reliable and helpful than those obtained by asking people to indicate which individual features are how important or what specific level is how desirable.

The results of this analysis will produce two types of marketing discoveries. First is the typical or average *preference ranking* or *rating of program* options, from the least to the most preferred. Second, and more important, is a set of what are called *utility functions,* which identify (1) the features that make the most difference to people's preferences and (2) the levels of those features that have the greatest effect. For example, results might show that in the context of other program features, location is the least important determinant of preference and choice of care experience is the most important. In addition, results might show that expectant mothers find obstetricians and family practitioners almost equally preferable but significantly downgrade all options that offer nurse midwives, or vice versa.

The combination of knowing which factors make the most difference and what level of each factor results in the greatest effect on preference should facilitate the design process enormously. The provider must decide whether it can or wishes to offer the option most attractive to the market, or rather offer something almost as good but more conducive to achieving mission and vitality objectives. Impractical mixes of features may be included in research in the interest of discovering preference patterns, but it may be just as wise not to ask about mixes that are impossible to deliver, since such options will have to be discarded even if they turn out to be preferred.

Markets are likely to prefer the program feature and level options that offer the best product in the most accessible place at the lowest price, although some interesting exceptions exist, especially regarding price. (People have been known to prefer an intermediate price to one lower, apparently believing that too low a price creates lower quality.) The provider may not be able or willing to offer a program that is superlative on all dimensions. By knowing the features and levels that have the greatest effect on preference, the provider can determine where necessary compromises can be made with the least negative impact on preference.

The techniques of LOGIT, conjoint, and functional analysis are chiefly used in the design of programs for new markets. Since most health care marketing deals with existing programs and markets, the provider should adapt these techniques to modifying existing programs. This can easily be accomplished through what might be called difference sensitivity analysis (DSA).

Difference Sensitivity Analysis

The mechanics of DSA are essentially similar to those of the analytical forms previously described. The difference is that instead of offering descriptions of program options in absolute terms, DSA describes features in terms of differences between one program and others. For example, instead of offering maternity package prices of $1500, $2000, and $2500, DSA would offer packages in which the options were: (1) $200 less, (2) equal to, and (3) $200 more than competing alternatives. Location options would be: (1) 5 minutes closer, (2) same distance, and (3) 5 minutes further away. When discrete rather than continuous features are involved, DSA would restate options in competitive terms: program A offers obstetricians, B offers family practitioners, and so on.

In DSA, selecting a representative set of options, offering them to a sample of potential and actual guests and other customers, and the analyzing of the results would be identical to the process used in LOGIT, conjoint, and functional analysis. The only change is that differences in competing alternatives rather than absolute levels of specific features would make up the alternative choices.

DSA selects the program features and levels so as to focus on distinctions and superiorities that the provider can offer compared to its competitors. Marketing must look not only to offer as attractive and satisfactory a guest or other customer experience as possible in an absolute sense, but one that is distinctive or superior (or both) on at least one significant feature. The distinctive or superior feature recognized by the market is likely to become important to and even determinant of choice, regardless of what abstract level of importance it might have. The DSA adaptation can focus on distinctions and superiorities that the organization can design into its offer and, then test the expected impacts on preference.

Tangible features may be enough for a successful marketing effort in selected circumstances. When persons are in a hurry to select a provider or are not highly motivated to consider alternatives, they may arrive at a preference on the basis of a few tangible features alone. (If opportunity and motivation are even lower, or if persons see no significant distinctions among their options, being the only known or most familiar option may suffice.) Being the closest available alternative, the one known to be open at a time care is needed, or the one provider known to offer a specific service may produce immediate preference.

At least three significant risks, however, accompany a tangible-feature marketing focus. First, the tangible features that determine choice may not be well identified. If even one significant feature is missing, the results of analysis may be misleading and design efforts may fail to produce as attractive and satisfactory a guest or other customer experience as intended. Second, the market segments to be attracted and satisfied may have such idiosyncratic preferences for features and levels that results fail to reveal any pattern on which to base successful design efforts. Third, and most critical, tangible features are only one of the bases that persons use to judge health care providers and programs. Both semitangible and intangible factors are likely to be influential as well.

Semitangible Perceptions

Several perceptions can best be described as semitangible. Features such as location, charges, provider categories, hours, and specific services offered are clearly tangible, designable, and describable in objective, factual terms. Semitangible perceptions are focused aspects of programs that can almost be designed in the same way as tangibles; however, patients and other customers judge and perceive these subjectively. For example, a judgment dimension such as convenience can be approached in terms of such tangible features as location, duration until appointment, and waiting time for care. A dimension such as costliness or reasonableness of price can be approached in terms of actual prices or how well physicians or technicians explain services and prices.

Whenever the provider already knows the tangible features that most determine judgments, the design phase can employ a semitangible feature approach. The essence of this approach is to research alternative mixes of features, not to discover the best or most preferred program option, but merely to determine which would be rated the most attractive or satisfactory on a single judgment dimension. Discovery results point to a given judgment dimension as important to preference and reveal that judgments on that dimension are explained and determined by perceptions of a few tangible features. The techniques of conjoint or functional analysis, LOGIT, or DSA, however, can be used to identify what program features would be most positively interpreted in terms of that dimension.

A marketer might show a series of location, hours, and appointment procedure options to a sample of prospects to learn which they would judge the most convenient. Such features would then be designed into the program offered by the organization. The expected result would not be stated in terms of overall preference ranking (evoked set), but rather in terms of a specific perception thought to influence preference (attribute set).

The judgment dimension of personal control or choice may be addressed through the relatively simple expedient of building a handful of patient and family choices into every patient experience. This may involve choices of diagnostic and therapeutic procedures in an informed-choice strategy or choices regarding timing and content of meals, mode of dress, and so on. Whenever known and clearly related tangible features for a given judgment dimension exist, the design process for semitangible perceptions is almost as simple as that based on tangible features.

Given the importance of achieving and maintaining a tangible distinction or semitangible superiority, it may be sufficient to focus on a single dimension, while seeking only parity on all or most others. Price, for example, is a dangerous feature for distinctions and superiorities, since it almost always entails a reduction in revenue per unit of service and thereby requires a substantial increase in volume just to achieve existing revenue outcomes. Location, services, and other tangible features may be difficult to change because of cost or regulatory constraints. Other tangible features may be easy to change, but concomitantly difficult to maintain a distinction or superiority in (e.g., hours, accepting charge cards).

In such circumstances, adopting a semitangible strategy and focusing design efforts on achieving and maintaining superiority in a specific judgment dimension may serve well in the marketing effort. Convenience clinics (urgicenters, minor emergency centers, immediate care centers), for example, have built their marketing strategies essentially on the dimension of convenience.[2] By combining extended hours and no-appointment-necessary procedures, these providers were able to establish a market niche between hospital emergency rooms and physicians' offices. If they are able to maintain positions as the convenient source of medical care, and as long as convenience is a major choice factor for enough people, they can survive and prosper without being better than other providers, perhaps even without being as good in such other dimensions as continuity.

In most cases, a semitangible design strategy attempts to develop a program offering that is equal or close to the competing market choices on most tangible and semitangible factors but significantly superior on one or two. By going through the list of judgment dimensions in Chapter 2, providers should be able to select which ones they can be at least equal on and which ones they can hope to achieve and maintain superiority. The semitangible approach to discovery should then identify which tangible features can be modified, added, or deleted with greatest effect on the selected intangible dimension.

As is true in all marketing, the focus of semitangible design must be on what customers perceive and how they interpret tangible features, not on how providers perceive and interpret them. To achieve quality and competence superiority in customers' minds, the provider may have to take steps that go far beyond meeting JCAH, Medicare, Medicaid, specialty board, or other professional notions of quality. This is not to deemphasize professional standards or definitions, but rather to emphasize the customer perspective as well. If customers are truly in error, misinformed, or otherwise interpreting tangible features incorrectly, providers may attempt to educate them accordingly. Until that education is successful, however, providers should respond to the ways people currently interpret features and arrive at preferences. It may make personnel in the organization feel good to be convinced that they offer the very best, but if the market is unconvinced, that feeling and the organization may be short-lived.

Intangible Perceptions

By definition, intangible factors in service, program, or provider selection exist only in customers' minds. In contrast to tangible or semitangible ones, intangible perceptions have no immediately manageable or designable response available. Intangible factors differ from semitangible ones only in *degree,* not in kind. Both involve persons' judgments and subjective perceptions that may or may not have any basis in reality. The chief difference between semitangible and intangible factors is the degree to which the tangible features that determine intangible judgments are known and related.

A judgment on continuity, for example, may be determined by whether receptionists, nurses, and physicians greet patients by name and are familiar with some aspect of their nonmedical lives. This may involve whether the employee can refer to prior shared experiences as easily as such tangible, easily manageable features as the patient's physical medical record. Judgments of competence may be influenced as much by whether a physician wears appropriate clothing, has diplomas on the wall, and asks the right questions as by results obtained or technical procedures followed.

From a design perspective, choices regarding tangible features should be dictated primarily by discovery results and management realities. The internal cost implications of adding, deleting, or modifying features should be readily estimable, together with their feasibility, acceptability, and so on. Management can usually make the design decisions involving tangible features, taking into account and incorporating suggestions by physicians, employees, patients, and families.

Choices regarding semitangible features are also within the traditional purview of managers. The more expensive and complex the specific feature involved, the more administration and governance may be involved; however, the narrow focus of semitangible design efforts usually warrants decisions and actions at the program management level. The degree of centralized vs. decentralized decision making, the scope of the marketing effort, and the cost and side effects of the design decisions will determine at what level specific design choices will be made.

Intangible judgments will probably be influenced by a variety of individual components from the guest or other customer experience. As "fuzzy" an intangible dimension as caring, for example, may be influenced by many interpersonal transactions—among physicians, guests, family, nurses, housekeeping staff, dietary aides, technicians, admitting clerks, volunteers, and others. Administrators and program managers may be hard-pressed to identify and implement designs that will systematically and effectively promote desired perceptions regarding intangible factors.

Ideally, the discovery phase of marketing will have supplied at least some insights into the sorts of tangible features that influence intangible judgments. For example, giving back rubs, responding quickly to call buttons, or explaining diagnostic and therapeutic procedures before and during their execution may be highly conducive to positive judgments of caring. Comfort may be affected by room temperature, how laundry is washed, noise levels, and so on. Typically, intangible judgments are affected by various often unrelated features, often not under the one manager's control. Several departments may be involved, or the features may be personality traits, behavior, and communication patterns of individual employees or physicians, and thus not readily "manageable."

The traditional model for the design phase is the *marketing mix*—product, place, and price—as was the case with marketing strategy. Pertinent questions include:

- What tangible features in each category will be viewed as most attractive and satisfactory by the guest and other customer markets targeted for attention?
- Which individual category of judgments along dimensions related to product/benefits, place/convenience, or price/costs would be the best focus for semitangible design efforts?
- What can the organization do to make its benefits, its access to service, and its charges more attractive and satisfactory to specific markets?

When it comes to intangible judgments, however, an alternative model is likely to work better: the cognitive script.[3]

The Cognitive Script

The cognitive script model of manageable features that affect intangible judgments is derived from a combination of psychology and theater. It is based on studies of how people experience, remember, and judge experiences in various situations, including restaurants, travel agencies, banks, and physicians' offices. It incorporates language and concepts derived from the stage: setting, props, characters, costumes, action, and dialogue.

Setting Features

The term *setting* in the cognitive script model covers all aspects of the provider's physical plant and campus that can influence how persons perceive the provider, whether in choosing a provider or in judging a guest or other customer experience. It includes the provider's location: Is it in a safe neighborhood? Is there parking available? Is it in a quality suburb or a declining slum? Is it convenient to travel and easy to find? In one of the few studies conducted on the effects of tangible features on intangible judgments, a suburban location was found to suggest greater competence, caring, and convenience to the public.[4]

Setting features also include how modern the facility appears to guests or customers. People seem to be impressed by a clearly new and modern facility, but not so much with a merely renovated one. The external appearance of buildings and grounds may suggest status to the status-sensitive person, a successful organization to the risk-sensitive person, or a competent or caring institution to another person.

The organization's internal setting is also an important influencer of intangible judgments. The decor can suggest bureaucratic rigidity or a homelike atmosphere, as in alternative birthing suites. The furniture may be comfortable, modern, in keeping with patients' preferences and expectations, or it may not. Colors may suggest sterility, promote calm, or provide reassurance. The sound levels, odors, and tactile aspects of the setting are all part of what are called *atmospherics* in marketing.[5]

Props

The tools and equipment used in delivering care or providing specific services also influence judgment. Is coffee served in plastic cups or china? Are electronic digital thermometers used, or manual mercury versions? Are tools and equipment strewn around the building for lack of storage space, becoming negative components of the setting? Do they work when used? From the guest's or other customer's perspective, the props used in the facility can produce strong impressions of competence or incompetence.

One can certainly argue that patients and other nonprofessional customers are not qualified to judge the appropriateness or significance of the tools and equipment used in rendering service. Unfortunately, they do make judgments about these "props," and it is in the best interest of the marketing provider to take this into account. All that is needed is the ability to appreciate the cognitive script aspects of the provider experience from the guest's or customer's point of view.

Characters

The personnel engaged in delivering care, whether personal, technical, or support services, also influence intangible judgments. Essentially, customers are likely to ask two questions, consciously or subconsciously, about the characters they interact with or notice.

1. Do they look like what they're supposed to be? Do physicians look like physicians, or do they appear too young or too old to be any good? Do nurses look like caregivers? Essentially, do people look right for their parts in the health care process, their roles in the delivery system?

2. Do they look like me? In an anxiety-producing provider selection situation, persons may be supersensitive to their conscious and unconscious biases. Minority patients may strongly prefer their peers as providers, whereas a majority population may question the competence of obvious foreigners. Women are increasingly indicating a preference toward female gynecologists. Patients and other customers may judge a provider's competence or compatibility by the "types" of other guests and visitors as well as by the characteristics of the employees or medical staff.

If props are a bothersome feature category, then the "characters" category will surely be unsettling. How can the personnel department carry out its function as if it were casting a play? How can any self-respecting provider cater to the public's prejudice and bigotry? How can an institution be an equal opportunity employer, or even keep its positions filled, if it has to worry about whether each applicant looks the part?

No clear or simple answers exist for these questions. It is simply an unavoidable reality that people make judgments based on the characters they relate to and otherwise notice in the provider environment. A provider may be able to take significant positive steps, such as recruiting female and minority employees to serve population segments who prefer them, or recruiting foreign-language physicians and employees to serve populations uncomfortable with English. Trying to influence the balance of patients, employees, and physicians or staff in light of recognized bigotry or uninformed prejudice is likely to be another matter altogether.

In recognition of persons' conscious and unconscious biases, the provider might undertake marketing communications efforts aimed at overcoming what might otherwise be the impressions given by characters. The backgrounds, qualifications, and accomplishments of physicians and employees could be publicized, for example, to counter what might be unconscious inferences of poor training in foreign professionals. Another approach is to ensure that majority physicians and employees treat their minority peers with special or at least clearly visible respect and esteem as a way of influencing patient and other customer attitudes.

Costumes

Another way of influencing the impressions made by the personnel delivering care is the use of "costumes." One can argue that persons should not make judgments based on anything as trivial as clothing, just as can be argued about props, setting, or characters. As is true for these other script features, however, costumes do influence customers' perceptions, both consciously and subconsciously. The very young or minority physician may look the part a little more if dressed for it.

One specific advantage that costumes can offer to guests and other customers is the opportunity to identify who works in the facility and what their responsibilities are. Being able to determine who is a nurse, a dietary aide, or technician can be helpful in directing a request to the right person. By contrast, not knowing whether a need or request should be expressed to one person or another can heighten a person's anxiety. Employees may object to the standardization or costs of uniforms, but they can be helpful in relations with guest and other customers.

Even other professionals are influenced by costumes. A "professional appearance" is likely to include what people wear as well as what they otherwise look like. In response to this, American Medical International's hospital employees are being garbed in standardized uniforms, much as airlines, hotels, restaurants, and other hospitality industries have done.[4]

51

Each organization must decide whether and how it will use costumes as a way of affecting the care process and relations with guests and other customers, as well as with physicians and employees.

Action

The "action" category in the cognitive script covers everything that guests and other customers do in the provider experience plus the many acts that physicians and employees perform. This includes such experiences as the admitting process, how long it takes, and how it is handled. It includes each test and treatment, how food is delivered, the types and amounts of activity programs made available, how rooms are cleaned and beds are changed—everything that happens to and in the sight of guests and other customers. Specific actions may suggest competence or caring, may deliver convenience, may protect privacy, and may allow choice; or they may not. Almost any judgment dimension outlined in Chapter 2 may be affected by action patterns.

Giving back rubs or other forms of therapeutic pampering may be more effective in communicating caring than words can convey. Having day-shift nurses introduce their evening counterparts may express continuity and caring, while adding to patient's psychological comfort and confidence. Answering call buttons promptly and responding to all guest requests are likely to influence judgments of courtesy and caring.

Dialogue

If "actions speak louder than words" in some ways, intangible judgments can be influenced by words, or "dialogue," at least as much as by actions. Dialogue covers everything said to guests and other customers, what they say and do not say in the care process, and everything they overhear. Competence and caring are likely to be communicated primarily by what providers say, although actions are critical as well. Reassurance, caring, confidentiality, continuity, courtesy, and control are provided largely through dialogue. Even impressions of convenience and cost can be influenced by whether and how long waits or charges are explained. Communicativeness is specifically a function of how dialogue between staff and guests or other customers is carried out.

How guests are addressed—as "dear," by first or last name, or without any salutation—can influence judgments of courtesy and respect as well as of caring. If providers know the guest's name and can refer to past encounters, this will influence perceptions of continuity. Choices have to be communicated if they are to be recognized and made. Physicians who ask patients what they think their problem is or whether they agree with the diagnosis are likely to find themselves rated higher in both competence and caring.

One of the patterns of responses that often emerges from guest and family surveys is that they do not get all the information they want or that they have a lot of trouble getting it. Ratings of providers on how informative they are tend to be low. To get higher ratings, providers often must volunteer information rather than wait to be asked or ask specifically if guests or family members have any questions. All this is part of managing the dialogue component of the cognitive script.

Scripting for Effect

One might appreciate how persons' judgments are influenced by features in the cognitive script categories, but marketing requires a way to identify exactly what to design into or out of the provider experience for desired effect. The most effective approach is likely to involve using the script categories as one checklist and the judgment categories as another. The marketer could then use the two checklists in a matrix format and organize discussions by script component: What could the institution do with setting features to reinforce, correct, or improve impressions of competence? What about caring, continuity, and so on? The matrix might also be tipped the other way: To reinforce, correct, or improve impressions of competence, how could the institution design or modify setting features? What about props, characters, costumes, and so on?

Such discussions can be carried out by administrators, department managers, or groups of employees. The *quality circles*[7] format can be used just as well for marketing purposes, focusing on reinforcing, correcting, or improving specific judgments by specific categories of guests and other customers. Some features in the setting and character categories are likely to require governing body approval or at least involve top administration. Some costume and prop features may be changeable at the department level. Employee groups and even individual employees may readily take action and dialogue steps.

The cognitive script and tangible categories may also focus on addressing human needs if a specific intangible judgment focus proves uncomfortable. Using Maslow's hierarchy of needs as a model, the provider could consider each script category to identify whether and how it might be used to respond better to persons' needs in the areas of:
- Physical survival and comfort: food, liquid, warmth, sleep
- Safety and security: reassurance, privacy, confidence that physical needs will be met and quality care will be given
- Belonging and love: caring, concern, continuity, feeling welcome, having needs responded to
- Esteem by self and others: courtesy, respect, convenience, confidentiality
- Achievement and self-actualization: ability to choose, participate in the care process, and recognize progress

- Knowledge and understanding: of one's disease or condition, of prognosis and treatment, of the ways the organization operates and how guests fit in
- Aesthetic appreciation: attractive surroundings, nice views

These basic need categories fit well with the judgment categories discussed in Chapter 2. They may be selected for attention through script categories or through the conventional marketing mix of product, place, and price. In most cases, no sure winners or ideas will always work. The focused imagination of administrators, managers, and employees is a better source of specific things to do than a book or even a marketing consultant. Internally developed design ideas also have the advantage of being much easier to implement.

Design Testing

Depending on the cost and degree of change involved in design ideas, the marketer may need to test some before implementation. It is always best to test design ideas after implementation to see if they have had any, and preferably a net positive, effect. Pretesting design ideas may take the form of opening up wider discussion or actual market testing on a small scale or temporary basis. Opening up a proposed change for wider discussion is clearly the easiest approach, but it may not always be best. Bringing in more persons may threaten the confidentiality of the idea and enable competitors to gain a jump. Other persons' involvement may introduce difficult conflicts and overly delay implementation. On the other hand, involvement by others can also introduce useful new insights and facilitate ultimate approval and implementation.

Market testing means actually trying out the change on a smaller scale or for a shorter period to see what happens. A guest relations idea might easily be tried out in one nursing unit or for one month, for example, in order to discover guest, physician, and employee reactions. One program or "product line" such as pediatrics or obstetrics might be chosen to test new decor or procedures (setting, action). New equipment or uniforms (props, costumes) might be tested in one facility of a multiinstitutional system before adoption by others is recommended.

The key in market testing is to use the discovery process to learn what the effects of such changes have been on guest and other customer attitudes. Marketing may need to modify guest satisfaction survey forms in order to pick up any shift in judgments engendered by a "script" change. Special surveys may be required to gauge physician, employee, or community reactions. Given the cost of such surveys, when special versions are needed, small samples and brief interviews may help reduce expenses, although they also limit the information that can be gained. Many changes will have to wait for regularly planned surveys.

The innovative provider taking patient attraction and satisfaction enhancement steps at frequent intervals should print guest satisfaction surveys in small quantities. A monthly or quarterly supply, if enough to ensure sufficient returns for valid conclusions, will enable the institution to print new forms in order to focus on specific steps taken. For example, if technicians come up with the idea of explaining to the patient and family satisfaction the tests and procedures they employ, then patient and family satisfaction forms might add a question about how communicative the staff has been and what specific experience most affected the communicativeness rating. Although not leading the guest, this would increase the likelihood that surveys will determine whether the change was noticed and how it affected guest or customer judgments.

When changes are developed out of a focus on a specific judgment dimension or human need, the evaluation of effect after a test or full implementation should clearly concentrate on that dimension or need. On the other hand, the evaluation should also note possible side effects. Other dimensions and needs should be included in feedback procedures to determine if either positive or negative (or both) effects on other guest, family, physician, employee, or public attitudes complement or mitigate the intended effects. Specific probes may be needed, which directly ask about a given change, to obtain specific relevant feedback. Such probes should always come at the end of the regular survey or questionnaire to avoid biasing the results.

Footnotes

1. Parker, B. and Srinivasan, V. "A Consumer Preference Approach to the Planning of Rural Primary Health Care Facilities." *Operations Research* 24:5 (Sep./Oct. 1976): 991.

2. Klegon, D. and Slubowski, M. "Marketing Ambulatory Care Centers." *Journal of Ambulatory Care Management* 8:3 (Aug. 1985): 18.

3. Smith, R. and Houston, M. "Script-Based Evaluation of Satisfaction with Services," in Berry, L. et al. (eds.) *Emerging Perspectives in Services Marketing.* Chicago: American Marketing Association, 1983, p. 59.

4. Neslin, S. "Designing New Outpatient Health Services: Linking Service Features to Subjective Consumer Perceptions." *Journal of Health Care Marketing* 3:3 (Summer 1983): 8.

5. Kotler, P. "Atmospherics as a Marketing Tool." *Journal of Retailing* 49:4 (1973): 48.

6. "Image Program Gives AMI Hospital Workers a New Look." *FAH Review* (Nov./Dec. 1984): 62.

7. Shaw, J. "Quality Circle Technique Aids Evaluative Criteria Process." *Hospital Progress* 63:8 (Aug. 1982): 49.

5. Delivering

The best strategic decisions and program designs are only as good as they can be translated into operations. The fourth phase of marketing requires that the provider implement the best-laid plans and intentions on a day-to-day basis. At this stage, marketing gives way to management. Ideally, a participative approach to discovering, deciding, and designing will have paved the way to effective delivering by ensuring that managers and employees both understand and support the objectives, strategies, and program specifics determined through these preceding phases.

From the guest's or other customer's point of view, what the organization delivers is the physical and personal experience that the institution offers. The obvious item delivered is the marketing mix of product (services, outcomes), place (location, hours, intake procedures), and price (charges, pain and discomfort, indignity). The combination of the physical plant, campus, furnishings, equipment, uniforms, and supplies (setting, props, costumes in cognitive script terms) constitutes the *physical experience.* The medical staff, employees, volunteers, other guests, and visitors with whom the guests and other customers interact (characters, action, dialogue) make up the *personal experience.*

Managing the Experience

The delivery of *product features* is relatively straightforward and familiar in health care administration. The range of services offered is a function of staff capabilities, equipment, supplies, and so on, coupled with whatever regulatory approval and financial assistance are required to develop new services. The quality of the product is the focus of certification programs and quality assurance efforts, which are well established in health care. Risk management and staff credentialing are other product-focused activities familiar to health care delivery.

Place features are equally familiar and manageable in most cases. The provider may offer satellite and mobile locations of service, such as computed tomography scans. It may extend or contract hours or modify intake procedures to facilitate use of its services. Regulatory and financial agencies may become involved if modifications are significant, but place features are still more or less under direct management control.

Price features are a little more complicated. Charges may still be under direct management control in most facilities, but the right to set them at whatever level is needed to ensure the bottom line has disappeared. Prospective reimbursement by government, competitive bidding, and rate control programs have taken this power away from managers. Moreover, the pain, discomfort, and other negative features of the guest experience are more likely to result from treatment of guests by personnel rather than from decisions that management makes. The challenge of managing personal interactions is discussed later.

The effects of program delivery management are relatively easy to monitor and evaluate. Ongoing or periodic surveys of guests, community, physicians, and employees allow marketing to track responses to any changes made in program features. The expenditure and revenue impacts of program changes are typically easy to gauge and are interrelated. Although the marketing terms of product, place, and price are relatively new in health care management, the basic concepts and techniques for managing them are thoroughly familiar, even as the rules of the game change.

Managing Physical Experience Delivery

The physical environment is also directly under management control. Design choices regarding facilities, decor, grounds, furniture, equipment, and supplies can be made and implemented with fairly precise estimates of costs. Managers can prepare budgets and have purchase orders and contracts signed to buy the necessary goods and services that will produce the changes designed for the physical environment. Some equipment purchases may still be under certificate-of-need (CON) control or may require the support of financial institutions for purchase. In general, however, the management of physical environment delivery factors is under administrative control.

Coupled with this more or less direct control and measurable cost is the unfortunate reality of indirect and difficult-to-measure effect. Data from community and guest surveys show significant sensitivity to physical environment factors, but not in as straightforward a way as to product, place, and price features. Physicians, employees, guests, and the public may react to changes in the buildings and grounds, to decoration and signs, and to uniforms and the equipment used for delivering care, but much of the reaction is likely to be subconscious. Thus, although the costs of implementing changes in the physical experience are more or less directly measurable, the impacts are not.

Managing Personal Experience Delivery

Management of the personal interactions of guests and other customers is a far more complex challenge than management of the marketing mix of program features or physical environment features. At the same time, it probably is the most important of the three categories of delivery features from a marketing perspective. Product, place, and price features are likely to be strongly determinant of market choices, but they are difficult to change in a dramatic way and competitors may readily copy them. Physical environment features are easier to change in most cases, but they are not as crucial to guest and customer attraction and satisfaction as are personal experience features.

Four basic components make up a systematic effort for managing personal experience:

1. Recruitment, screening, and selection
2. Orientation, training, and ongoing education
3. Leadership and observation
4. Performance evaluation, recognition, and reward

Management should use all four in an integrated marketing and human resources program that covers employees, medical staff, and volunteers. Any one of the components may be enough in some cases, but the ideal program will take advantage of the synergistic effects of managing all four.

Recruitment, Screening, and Selection

Obtaining the right personnel initially is clearly the most effective first step in managing, that is, getting things done through other persons. Health care should have a head start in this regard, since it should attract persons trained or at least committed to serving others. The religious hospital or long-term-care institution should tend to attract those with some sort of spiritual or psychological commitment to religious values. The recruitment, screening, and selection functions of human resource management should aim at attracting, identifying, and hiring (or adding to the medical staff and volunteer staff) those who have the proper personalities and commitments.

Managers should use some combination of personality testing and personal interview to gauge the values and priorities that motivate applicants, in addition to reviewing their qualifications. Interest in people as opposed to ideas or material values should be great in almost anyone who is to work in the facility, unless interaction with others is not a substantial part of the job. The more clearly and consistently the provider's own values are spelled out, the easier it will be to determine how consistent prospective members' values are with them.

If a bright side exists to the decline in inpatient utilization that began in the early 1980s, it may be that hospitals do not have the types of staff shortages common when utilization was higher and growing every year. Consequently, hospitals should spend the time needed to determine the values and priorities of prospective employees, medical staff, and volunteers. The individuals who form the hospital organization and create the personal experience delivered may change, but the system of values that drives the facility should be relatively constant. This is best ensured by making certain that the persons with the proper values are the ones attracted to the hospital.

The same opportunity exists regarding medical staff. With the surplus of physicians and declining numbers of hospitals, individual institutions can and must be more selective in medical staff development. New motivations and criteria apply: prudent case management tendencies, ability to work with others, commitment to good patient relations, as well as technical expertise. In addition, commitment to or at least consistency with the institution's values, mission, and vitality should be an important consideration in choosing medical staff members.

Nursing homes need to recruit persons who are comfortable dealing with physically and mentally declining residents, who are committed to service and professional quality, and who are basically caring individuals. Sensitivity to psychological, social, and spiritual needs and to family as well as resident concerns is essential in such employees, for quality of care as well as for marketing reasons.

This form of *character management* is at least as important as obtaining those who "look the part" or are compatible with the expectations and wishes of patients and other customers. It places a high value on the personnel function and suggests that marketing give some input into human resources management. This latter suggestion becomes even more important as the remaining three components are discussed.

Orientation, Training, and Ongoing Education

Once the right personnel have been recruited, selected, and hired or added to the staff, management must supply them with the information, motivation, and experience that will enable and encourage them to function most effectively. In addition to traditional orientation, training, and education aimed at technical skills, quality, productivity, and efficiency, attention should focus on organizational values and marketing.

Managers should inform employees and medical staff members about the impact of their behavior on guest or customer attraction and satisfaction and about expectations that they contribute positively to these marketing goals. Physicians should be assisted in their efforts toward attracting and satisfying their own patients and referrals.

Values orientation, training, and education efforts are especially important and appropriate in religious health care. The organization at least should have clearly stated values relative to:
- The essential worth and dignity of individual human life
- The value and importance of employee effort and work
- Management's commitments to human and religious values in its relations with employees, guests, and physicians
- Organizational commitments to service, the community, the poor, or any particular group
- Organizational commitments to colleagues in the health care system
- Organizational commitments to excellence in management, marketing, operations, and so on

Management should communicate such values to prospective and current members as clearly and strongly as possible.

St. Joseph Hospital, Kansas City, MO, uses one approach to clarifying and communicating values. The hospital created a Values Constitution, which stated the values of the hospital and its sponsoring religious institute, as well as the implications of those values in terms of behavior. After each value, the constitution lists actions that members of the hospital organization strive to perform as part of their day-to-day relations with each other, patients, and the community. Copies of the constitution are given to employees, volunteers, auxiliary members, and medical staff, as well as to patients, families, and friends. Such clearly stated and published commitments represent promises that all hospital members make to each other and those they serve.[1]

Leadership and Observation

This category of contributions to delivery covers most of conventional operations management. It includes what managers say and do in efforts to encourage and enable organization members to fulfill value commitments and achieve marketing and management goals. It includes the setting and enforcement of both formal and informal standards and day-to-day observation of and interaction with employees, medical staff, and others. Most importantly, it includes leadership and example-setting by management.

A well-established maxim in service marketing states that the way management treats employees becomes the way employees treat customers. One could also say that the way managers treat customers becomes the way employees treat customers. The administrator who guides a lost visitor, regularly visits the patient units, and helps out in patient care is showing what is important and getting the message across in a way that mere words cannot. The best move I ever made in my own brief career in hospital administration was to remove the chair from my office so that I had to take a "walking around" approach to management.

The most clearly and cleverly stated values will mean nothing if managers do not demonstrate them consistently and visibly in their day-to-day relations with all members of the health care organization and those it serves. Health care personnel must express organizational values with observable behavior as well as with verbal philosophical commitments, and managers must demonstrate and monitor that behavior. Ideally, employees will monitor each other as well. This becomes more likely if management's example in relations with employees and patients is a clear and constant demonstration of the organization's stated values.

Performance Evaluation, Recognition, and Reward

In addition to everyday example, management demonstrates the importance of stated values through the ways it evaluates, rewards, and recognizes the contributions of members. If rewards go to those who play internal politics most effectively, then organizations are demonstrating the priority value of playing politics, regardless of what they say are their true values. If rewards go only for financial contributions, then that is what the organization values. If recognition is given to those who provide quality care and respond effectively to human needs, then those are the important values.

Positive feedback from management and preferably from peers should be both frequent and consistently focused on what the organization truly values. Once-a-year performance evaluations and merit raises are far too infrequent and too little to serve as an effective component of delivery. A risk always exists that positive feedback will become so frequent and automatic that it will lose its meaning, but that is rarely the case. As marketing contributions, that is, additions to the provider's ability to attract and satisfy patients, become valued, they should be identified, recognized, and rewarded, in the same way as contributions to quality, productivity, and efficiency.

Marketing Circles

A day-to-day management approach with great promise in marketing seems to be marketing circles.[2] The mechanics of such circles are borrowed directly from quality circles, although the focus is shifted to attracting and satisfying patients and other customers. The idea is to incorporate employees directly in the organization's marketing effort and recognize their contributions to that effort by giving them the power to make their own changes in pursuit of marketing objectives.

As with any marketing effort, marketing circles begin with the discovering step, focusing attention on guest and customer feedback from systematic surveys, letters of praise, or complaints. These are analyzed and summarized as appropriate for each group of employees that forms a circle. Some providers may form circles in employee categories: nurses, housekeepers, dietary aides, admitting clerks, and so on. Others may organize employees around product or patient experience categories (emergency room, pediatrics, rehabilitation), grouping employees from all categories who create the patient experience in a particular program. The two approaches may be mixed as necessary to keep the size of the group within manageable limits (no more than 15 members, preferably 6 to 10).

Once circles are formed and supplied with feedback, they discuss the objective features under their, or at least organizational, control that can be used to improve patients' and other customers' attraction and satisfaction. A useful approach to this task involves a *features-feelings matrix*. As was discussed about the intangible opinions or feelings persons use to judge alternative choices and actual experience, the feelings part of the matrix might involve a list of judgment dimensions: competence, caring, convenience, continuity, cost, comfort, confidence, courtesy, control, commitment, communicativeness, cleanliness, and conviviality.

Discussion would focus on the question: "What can we say and do that will reinforce or improve what patients and other customers conclude about us in each of these categories?" A logical list of features to complete the matrix would be the cognitive script categories of setting, props, characters, costumes, action, and dialogue. Discussion might start with each script feature in order and ask: "How can we use that factor to reinforce or improve people's judgments regarding one or more of these judgment dimensions?" Another option would be to start with each judgment dimension in order and ask: "How can we reinforce or improve the way people judge us in terms of (competence, for example) using one or more of the six feature categories?"

If employees are uncomfortable or uncertain about focusing on the 10 judgment dimensions, Maslow's hierarchy of needs may be an effective substitute. Circle participants would review their list of features, looking for ways to respond to basic human needs:

1. Physical comfort, survival, feeling good
2. Safety and security, peace of mind
3. Belonging needs, feeling welcome, cared about
4. Esteem, respect, feeling valued by others and oneself
5. Actualization, feelings of achievement
6. Knowledge and understanding, feeling well-informed
7. Enjoying sights, sounds, tastes, and so on

Since many aspects of patient experience threaten Maslow-type feelings, considerable discussion should probably focus on the question: "What can we do or say to keep people's feelings of (physical comfort, safety, belonging, esteem, achievement) from being threatened or harmed any more than necessary?"

In most cases, the ideas that emerge from marketing circle discussions can be implemented by the participants, without investment or involvement by management or other groups. When ideas go beyond what can so readily and immediately be implemented, management becomes involved. In larger facilities, employee, department head, and administrative circles may work together toward the same goals. The ideas emerging from employee groups tend to enhance implementation and enthusiasm.

Marketing circles are a form of recognition and reward, since they accord employees the power to control some of their activities. As a second source of recognition and reward, these circles use the feedback from guests and other customers. For best effect, patient surveys and any other ongoing feedback mechanisms should be flexible enough to use in looking for response to ideas that have been implemented, with circles checking to see if anyone has noticed any change, and if so, what they think about it. It is useful to reproduce survey or other feedback forms on copying machines or print them in small numbers rather than be locked into a single form for years.

When checking specific responses, questions should not ask: "What do you think of (the action taken or change made)?" Rather, they should ask persons first to rate their feelings on the judgment dimension or Maslow need category intended to be affected, then to indicate what caused them to answer as they did. This will indicate any effect on overall opinion and determine whether the changes made accounted for some part of any opinion effects. Only if no sign of effect is detected in this manner should a question ask directly about a specific change. Even then, responses should be viewed suspiciously, because direct questions tend to bias results.

Systematic feedback should provide a *customer pull* effect that complements the *management push* effect of orientation and training, leadership and observation, and performance evaluation. It also provides its own reward and recognition effect, giving employees a sense of accomplishment independent of management. The combination of marketing circles and systematic feedback also serves to maintain a high degree of employee sensitivity to their importance in and contributions to organizational marketing efforts.

Internal Marketing and Religious Values

Marketing and religion obviously are not the same. Conventional marketing intentions of putting the competition out of business may often be incompatible with religious values. On the other hand, a great area of compatibility exists between religious values and marketing, as illustrated through suggested marketing strategies. Treating employees as important human beings with intrinsic dignity and worth makes good marketing sense. According the same to guests and other customers is even more clearly a sensible marketing approach. The golden rule can serve as a guide to guest and customer relations just as well as to all human interaction.

From a management point of view, the key to marketing effectiveness lies in the behavior of all members of the organization. When marketing sensitivity combines with personal and religious values to produce guest and customer experiences that are attractive and satisfactory, the provider should succeed. If they produce experiences distinctly superior to what competitors offer and deliver, as judged by guests, physicians, and others who make health care decisions, a possibility always exists that competitors may be forced out of business. It makes little sense to do less deliberately or do it less well to protect the competition.

Providers that hire, train, manage, and reward persons with strong personal and religious values consistent with the provider's own values probably will prosper in today's competitive health care environment, not despite but because of such values. Those in the health business for the sole purpose of making profit are likely to communicate that motivation to their employees and guests, with negative results, at least in the long run. Although commitments to the poor and to community service, even if unprofitable, put religious health care at a business disadvantage, religious values do not put providers at a marketing disadvantage. Living out religious values in decision, design, and delivery should contribute to the marketing success and survival of religious health care organizations.

Footnotes

1. Lazio, M. "A New Beginning." *Together* (published by St. Joseph Hospital, Kansas City, MO) 6:1 (Jan. 1985): 9.

2. MacStravic, R.S. "Marketing Circles in Practice Development." *Journal of Professional Services Marketing* 2:1 (Fall 1986).

6. Describing

Describing what the organization can offer its customers completes the five-step marketing process. In marketing terminology, this step is referred to as *promotion,* but a more appropriate term would be *marketing communication.* It includes all communications to prospective and current customers that have a primary or even secondary marketing purpose. The term *advertising* would apply if the dictionary definition were used, but advertising has come to be associated with a narrow focus on public media. Marketing communication, or describing, goes far beyond that.[1]

The purpose of describing is to affect the minds of the persons who receive marketing communications. The ultimate purpose is almost always expressed in terms of behavior, such as use of services, working at the facility, or joining its medical staff, but the proper objective in designing marketing communications is the mental status of selected communications targets. Thus the most important step in describing is to specify the persons who should receive the descriptions.

Targets

Given the complexity of health care decisions and the various decisions that providers might wish to influence, many possible targets might be specified for any particular description strategy, campaign, or message. In marketing communication, a *strategy* is a comprehensive set of campaigns aimed at whatever sets of targets the provider wishes to reach and covering whatever sets of knowledge, attitudes, and behaviors it wishes to influence. A *campaign* is an organized set of messages aimed at a particular set of targets and intended to achieve a particular purpose. A *message* is a single communication that may be repeated several times or delivered through various methods to a particular set of targets.

Since strategies, campaigns, and messages might be used for various reasons, targets might include potential and current guests, donors, medical staff members, employees, employers, legislators, regulators, and financiers; that is, anyone whose mental status and behavior the provider wishes to influence. The most effective basis for developing communications is a precise and complete specification of (1) who the targets are; (2) where they live, work, or otherwise can be reached; (3) what is currently in their minds; (4) what sources of information they rely on; and (5) how their mental status affects their behavior.

The discovery step in marketing is responsible for supplying this kind of intelligence. In some cases, the decision step identifies targets first; through characteristics such as place of residence, health status, employment status, and potential contribution to the provider's mission or vitality, it specifies who should be targets for communication. Then discovery conducts the appropriate research to learn what is needed to develop an effective description approach. In other cases, discovery comes first and targets are selected based on the persons most likely to be easily and effectively reached and influenced. In any case, once targets are specified, marketing should discover four "state of mind" factors as the next step in developing communications.

States of Mind

General readiness. The first state of mind is the general state of readiness to act and to choose one of several competing options. Depending on the circumstances, this might involve recognition of a problem, perception of a need, or any other state of mind that motivates a person to begin considering taking some action. Motivating potential patients to recognize symptoms or perceive the need for a check-up are examples. Because many persons have undiscovered hypertension, diabetes, and arterial disease, communications might be aimed at motivating them to seek out screening services. Except for routine and habitual behavior, persons presumably must feel the *need* to take some action before they will consider and make choices.

Communications might be aimed at those people who recognize a given problem or perceive a given need or at their definition of the problem or need. In a prepaid insurance plan, for example, marketing efforts might seek to persuade members that a common cold is not amenable to medical intervention. In other circumstances, efforts might be aimed at influencing what problems and needs people define as medical/health situations rather than "wait-until-it-goes-away" situations. In marketing terms, industrial advertising might be used to increase total demand for a good or service. Then everyone who sells such goods and services will share a greater volume of business.

Evoked Set Responses. The second state of mind is the set of responses persons call to mind when they recognize a problem or perceive a need. This evoked set of responses involves not only what people call to mind but also the order of precedence or preference in which they call them. As discussed in Chapter 3, the five positions are (1) only known response, (2) top-of-mind response, (3) acceptable alternative, (4) best response, and (5) only acceptable response.

People with low levels of motivation, little information, and little time may either go immediately to the *only response* they know or, if they know of none, look until they find one. A stranger may look in the Yellow Pages or ask the first person encountered where the nearest source of medical care or the nearest hospital is located never bothering to look for other options. This might occur in an emergency when no time is available to reflect on choices. It might also occur with a routine need such as for a preemployment physical; the person would simply not consider it important enough to look for more than one alternative. Communications in such circumstances would be aimed at making the hospital or a specific program widely known and widely listed in directories, billboards, and other media that people might use.

In similar circumstances, if persons have low motivation or little time to consider alternatives but are aware of more than one option, they tend to go for the most familiar or *top-of-mind option.* They have no real preference among their alternatives and see no reason to form a preference; they simply lean toward the better known or more recognized option. Communications in such circumstances would be aimed at making one provider more widely known, using publicity, advertising, and any other appropriate communications methods. Both only known and top-of-mind positions are better than being unknown or below the top, but they are essentially weak positions subject to being superseded by the best response or the only acceptable response position.

Selection of a response often follows a two-stage process. If the person evokes several alternatives for consideration, the first tendency is to reduce that number to two or three, rarely more. To select a limited number of *acceptable alternatives,* all options that have significant negative attributes (e.g., too far away, too expensive) are eliminated. The person may view those that remain as roughly equivalent. Without strong positive distinction or superiority to single out one choice, two or three may be seen as acceptable. Getting at least that far in the selection process is better for the provider than being evoked and rejected, but not as good as being rated best.

Whenever persons have the time and motivation to consider competing options and arrive at a preference, they are likely to decide one option is the *best choice.* Their reasons for considering one as the best may vary and differ significantly from what professionals would consider appropriate. The provider placed as the best choice is in a stronger position than any providers placed below. In normal circumstances, persons will seek out the best, although barriers might arise. If all beds are filled, if the physician recommends another provider, or if a service is needed that the best hospital does not offer, then the person might go elsewhere. Communications aimed at achieving a best choice position must give targets enough evidence and arguments, in terms of what they will use to judge options, to select one provider as the best.

If a position as best choice is strong enough and other options are rated far below it, a provider may enjoy a position as the *only acceptable choice.* This differs from being the best choice only in the degree of preference, but it is a stronger position to hold. Prospective patients or referring professionals would delay placement rather than seeking another nursing home; they would lobby for the only proper hospital to offer a service not currently available rather than accept the idea of going elsewhere. A patient whose physician recommended another facility would insist on the only proper one; one whose physician lacked privileges at the only proper hospital would switch physicians. Communications aimed at achieving such a position must identify significant distinctions and superior characteristics that make other options unacceptable.

Attribute Set Judgments. The third state of mind of targets is the set of criteria that they use in judging and selecting among competing options, together with the perceptions they have of such options on those criteria. This attribute set of judgment dimensions and specific beliefs only applies if preference is involved, that is, only to situations where targets select acceptable options, a best or only proper option. To be positioned as best or only proper choice, a provider must be perceived as distinctive or superior in dimensions that targets consider important. The provider must be able to speak to targets in terms that they understand and cite information that will affect their preferences. It does no good to describe what the provider is proud of unless that information is also significant to targets.

Information Source Responses. The fourth state of mind factor that discovery should learn about targets is the sources of information that they have used in the past and rely on in the present. For communications to be effective, they must not only speak to targets in terms they understand and consider significant, but must also reach those targets and be heard. Knowing what sources of information have influenced targets' knowledge and attitudes in the past will also help gauge the strength of their states of mind.

In general, the strength of people's beliefs and attitudes vary greatly with the sources of information on which they were based. In descending order of strength, such sources are likely to be:

1. Personal experience; such as being a guest, employee, or volunteer in the facility and knowing the experience by having undergone it
2. Vicarious experience; seeing the experience of a family member or friend and knowing the experience by observing it
3. Specific comments made by others in response to questions, their recounted experiences, advice by presumed authorities when requested
4. General comments, conventional wisdom, reputation of the organization based on casual stories of other persons' experience or what others have heard
5. Published reports, media stories, and features that qualify as news in persons' minds
6. Advertising or other information known to originate from the organization

Putting it last is not meant to denigrate the importance of advertising, but to put it in perspective. Ads may be the fastest and most effective way of communicating specific information regarding a new program or development or significant changes in the facility. The high degree of control offered by advertising, over both who receives messages and what those messages contain, makes this method particularly useful for many purposes. On the other hand, given the importance of personal experience, both directly through the first two sources listed and indirectly through the next two, no provider should expect to succeed through advertising in generating opinions that are much different from how actual experience is judged.

Communications Options

Five basic channels are available through which marketing communications may be transmitted to their intended targets:

1. Personal contact includes communication on a one-to-one basis, through speeches and programmed discussions, in person, by phone, or through personal correspondence.
2. Direct delivery includes messages sent through the mail or delivery services rather than through public media.
3. Advertising covers all use of paid time and space in public media, including radio and television, newspapers, and magazines.
4. Publicity includes everything that public and private media say about the provider, with or without its help.
5. Word-of-mouth communications include all solicited and unsolicited comments that persons make about the provider to

their family, friends, acquaintances, and strangers.

Personal contact is most useful when the persons doing the contacting can use charisma or interaction with their targets to enhance the effect of messages. Physicians and other authorities can be more influential this way. Sales representatives can use personal contact with employers to carry out market research and tailor their message to their targets. Personal contact by phone and mail can thank physicians for referrals, check on satisfaction, and otherwise spread goodwill as well as deliver specific messages. When the right persons are used with the right targets, personal contact can be the most effective means of transmitting messages, although it tends to be the most expensive as well.

Direct delivery has the great advantage of offering total control over who receives messages. Through selected mailing or delivery lists, providers can ensure that everyone they wish to reach and no one else actually gets a particular message. They cannot be as certain that everyone who receives it and only those intended will read the message, but control is almost as great as with personal communication. Direct delivery also is likely to be more acceptable to most audiences, as compared to media advertising, for example. On the other hand, it may be dismissed as "junk mail." Since written communications, multicolor brochures with pictures, audiotapes, and even videotapes can be used in direct delivery, the range or cost of communications in this category has no limit.

Media advertising offers almost total control over communications content but substantially less over targets. Some radio stations and special interest magazines or newspapers may offer narrow population segments, but the chances of them matching perfectly the intended audience for a given message are slim. Advertising also suffers from a high degree of "noise" and competition for attention and tends to have low credibility for most audiences. Good advertising, however, can be very effective for specific purposes. Unfortunately, it can also be very expensive and may take a long time to be effective.

Publicity should be substantially less expensive, although having good media relations, sponsoring newsworthy events, and maintaining a public relations staff involve considerable expense. Stories in public or private publications or over radio or television tend to have higher credibility than advertisements, but they are far more difficult to control. Both content and timing of messages are subject to the publisher's wishes. Moreover, many messages, including discussions of distinctions and superiorities compared to competitors, probably will not be accepted for publicity.

Word-of-mouth communications are probably the most effective means of general public communication and in most cases are free. They are easily the most difficult to control, however, and require constant attention for best effect. The management of word-of-mouth communications should be part of every provider's marketing strategy, although relatively few practice such management.[2] Religious health care, with its not-for-profit nature and community service mission, may benefit more naturally from word-of-mouth contributions. In word-of-mouth, maximum effectiveness only comes from effective discovery, decision, design, and delivery support, but this is true for all marketing communications.

Tangibles and Intangibles

Basically two categories of perceptions influence how people judge competing provider options and place them in their evoked set of choices. As noted previously, tangible perceptions involve awareness and beliefs regarding objective, factual attributes of the provider and its particular programs. Important tangibles are likely to include location of the provider, the specific programs and services it offers, hours of availability, and charges. In some circumstances, distinctions on such attributes will dictate preference; for example, if only one provider offers maternity or if one of its programs is the only one available when someone wants immediate care. If its charges are lower, the provider may win in a competitive bidding situation with employers or insurance companies.

When tangible factors alone will dictate choice, communications need only present the facts in an objective, educational format. Since they can reach many persons faster, publicity and advertising might be more effective than personal communications or word-of-mouth to transmit messages regarding changes in tangible features. Advertising of specific tangible information is also more likely to be believed, at least when compared to intangible claims. Such advertising is also less likely to arouse concern among physicians, employees, peers, and the public, as long as it discusses only the organization and does not make comparisons to other competitors.

Intangible factors cover the entire list of factors discussed in detail in Chapter 4. Any communications regarding competence, convenience, caring, commitment, and so forth share the challenge of how to be believable. Because such factors are intangible, that is, exist only in the mind of the beholder, anyone can claim them without the recourse to verification associated with tangible factors. People are used to claims of intangibles from all kinds of advertisers, from used car salesmen to cigarette ads. They are likely to dismiss most, especially if claims are not consistent with what word-of-mouth reputations suggest.

The essence of effective marketing communications rests on the ability to create perceptions in the minds of targets that the provider is distinct or superior in some way that makes it the best or only proper choice for particular problems and needs. It is particularly challenging, both practically and ethically, to communicate distinctions and superiorities regarding intangible dimensions. Three different approaches might be used: direct claims or indirect assertions by the provider, testimonials from individuals or groups, and tangible evidence with or without claims.

Direct claims may be made in various ways: "We Care!" "Come to _____ Hospital for Caring and Convenience," "Our Maternity Program Lets You Decide," and so on. In general, such claims are likely to be accepted at face value by only the most gullible persons, who might then accept similar claims by competitors the next day. If such claims are supported by direct, tangible evidence, such as maps or instructions showing the provider's convenient location, specific examples of choices offered in services, or nurses expressing their care by giving back rubs, persons are more likely to believe them. It is theoretically possible through visual associations, such as showing pictures of friendly but concerned maternal-looking nurses, to strengthen verbal claims. The combination of *claim, evidence,* and *association* is likely to be more effective than any one or two alone.

Indirect assertions are typically made in the form of slogans or mottoes, such as "The Best Care Comes From The Heart" (Sacred Heart General Hospital, Eugene, OR) and "Health-Healing-Hope" (St. John's Hospital, Longview, WA). Such slogans may reinforce and resensitize targets to perceptions or reputations that already are present but are unlikely to be persuasive alone. These slogans are also abetted in their impact by visual or aural associations. They are enhanced even further if some form of evidence is supplied either by the provider or through word-of-mouth communications.

Testimonials by individuals may take the form of stories of good outcomes of care, good guest experiences, or directly quoted comments by satisfied, pleased, or delighted customers. Any testimonials on outcomes may run afoul of either ethical objections, such as by the American Medical Association, or legal objections, such as by the Federal Trade Commission (FTC), if outcomes are not demonstrably typical. Outcome discussions may raise expectations in other patients that lead to malpractice suits if unfulfilled. Testimonials regarding good guest experiences are less troublesome, although the FTC may object if they are not typical. Directly quoted comments are subject to the same limitation, but an indirect alternative exists: publishing the names and phone numbers of satisfied guests and other customers (with their permission) and suggesting that interested targets contact them.

Group testimonials may be used in the form of publishing the results of opinion polls. For example, the provider could publish the overall results of guest satisfaction surveys. Organizations should ensure that such results are statistically reliable and valid and that they are described accurately. Community survey results may also be used to show how others view the provider. The provider may even publish comparisons if surveys have asked persons to compare or rate competing providers separately, although this may invite a comparison war. Besides, it is unclear how many persons would be swayed by learning that 60 percent of the local population prefer Hospital A to Hospital B.

Tangible evidence may be transmitted with or without its intended intangible claim. If discovery has determined that particular targets view some specific tangible feature as a sign of some intangible characteristic, then the organization may simply communicate the tangible fact, relying on the audience to reach the proper conclusion. Describing how the institution's nurses answer call buttons in an average of 45 seconds may persuade audiences that the institution's staff is responsive or even caring, and committed. Indicating that 93 percent of staff physicians are board certified may persuade audiences that the organization is competent. Listing services offered may persuade audiences that the hospital or nursing home is a comprehensive or full-service institution.

To ensure that targets reach the intended conclusion, the provider may insert it in the communication. Rather than begin the message with a claim of competence, convenience, caring, and so forth, organizations could include all their evidence first, then make a claim at the end, such as, "We think you'll agree that our nurses are especially caring." The best way to decide whether evidence alone or evidence plus conclusion works best is to pretest the message (see Chapter 2). Of course, this applies to any message, regardless of the content approach used.

Basic Message Content

Five components should be used in designing most messages:
1. Grabber—headline, attention getter
2. Theme—conclusion audience should reach
3. Body—arguments, claims, evidence, and associations that will lead audiences to the intended conclusion
4. Hook—response requested of audience if they reach the intended conclusion
5. Signature—logo, name of sponsor, or slogan to link message content with the right organization

Grabber. The grabber may be words, sounds, pictures, action, or any combination of these, depending on the medium. The effective grabber will gain the attention of the intended audience in the midst of today's vast clutter of messages. The first task of any message is to gain the attention of its intended audience. Failure in this task guarantees that whatever may be contained in the rest of the message will be wasted.

The grabber in practice may involve a sound (siren, baby crying, auto horn, shout), a picture (well-known or attractive person, a baby, someone who resembles the intended audience), or words (Hey You! Under Stress? A New Service for You!). The grabber can be used to gain the attention of precisely the audience that should pay attention to the message: "New in Town?" for a message concerning a physician referral service, for example. It might be based on an appeal to curiosity: "It Was A Dark and Stormy Night . . . " to begin a story related to emergency medical services. A fear appeal might be used: "Are Your Children Safe?" for a discussion of immunization. A benefit might be suggested: "Faster Care When You Need It" for a convenience care program. A nursing home message might begin with the headline: "Has Mother Become Another Child?"

As with all parts of good messages, marketing should design grabbers with care and test them before use. If pretesting is impractical, alternative forms of the same message, with different grabbers, may be used to gauge which works best. Since persons vary and different segments might be the intended audiences for particular messages, no surefire grabbers exist. Experience over time, aided by systematic pretesting and careful evaluation, will promote learning and improve effectiveness of all parts of message design.

Theme. The theme is the specific conclusion or idea that audiences are supposed to reach as the result of being exposed to the message. The starting point of all messages should be this theme, even though the grabber typically begins the message. What should the audience be aware of, believe, feel, or do as the result of experiencing the message? Health educators are familiar with designing educational experiences based on measurable behavior objectives. The same logic applies to communications experiences of all types, including marketing messages.

Marketing should usually choose themes carefully and state them clearly before developing any other part of the message and before discussing media selection. Themes should be based on what is known from discovery about what targets know, feel, and do and what motivates their choices and behavior. Themes may address what is already in targets' minds, to reinforce and resensitize them to established beliefs and feelings. Themes may strive to place new knowledge, beliefs, or attitudes in persons' minds, establishing these where no or only weak content exists. In some cases, themes may aspire to replacing what is in targets' minds, shifting beliefs and preferences away from existing content.

Generally, it takes less content (i.e., fewer messages, fewer repetitions) in each message to reinforce than to establish, and less to establish than to replace. In most cases, marketing should consider this when choosing targets and objectives. The same message might be used for many purposes, but the content, exposure, and number of repetitions must be adequate to fulfill its most difficult purpose. The theme, when contrasted to the known state of mind of identified targets, will indicate how much of a challenge is being accepted and how much of an investment is likely to be needed.

Body. The body covers the main content of the message, that is, everything that is not a grabber, hook, or signature. Its design should lead targets to the intended conclusion as effectively and efficiently as possible. If a few words or sentences will do it, then that is what should be used. If several paragraphs are required, then the body may be long. No limit on length can be arbitrarily applied; messages should be long enough to make audiences reach the intended conclusion, and no longer. If the body content is interesting enough, audiences will stay with it. If it is not relevant or attention grabbing, it makes no difference how short it is.

Hook. The hook represents a specific behavioral response that the message asks the audience to make: call a number, write a letter, or send in a coupon. A direct hook asks audiences to do something that the sponsor can measure as a way of gauging the message's effect. Slightly varying hooks may be used to check which message drew how much response, such as different phone numbers, names to write, or PO box numbers. The theme may go no further than necessary to cause audiences to make the hook response. That response would then lead to more messages and subsequent conclusions, such as when audiences call for more information, a pamphlet, or a recorded message. If the message leads them further, the hook may involve calling for an appointment or otherwise seeking a specific service.

Indirect hooks are responses that audiences are asked to make but the sponsor cannot measure. These hooks, however, involve audiences more in the message and enhance its effect. Persons might be asked to look in the mirror, step on a scale, or consciously examine some part of their body or its function. The message would supply the motivation to do so and the information about what to look for, then suggest a subsequent response. Indirect hooks are often used to increase sensitivity to a known problem, perhaps with subsequent impact on service use. The marketer may gauge their effect by asking persons who come to a physician's office, hospital clinic, or nursing home why they did so. An indirect hook should engage the audience in a behavioral response rather than mere passive reception. Any response will tend to greatly enhance the effect of the message.

Signature. As its name suggests, the signature is typically the last part of a message. Its purpose is to link the message, and especially the conclusion or theme, clearly and permanently with the provider sponsoring the message. Failure to establish such a link will mean failure to benefit from the rest of the message's effect. The signature normally contains the name of the sponsor, perhaps its address and phone number, plus a clearly identifiable logo and maybe a slogan or motto. It should be placed and designed so as to ensure that audiences recognize it along with the rest of the message and connect the theme to the right provider. Even if the theme requests a general response, such as seeing a physician or receiving an immunization, the provider's signature should stand out, if only to promote familiarity and image.

As with all parts of marketing messages, marketing should test and evaluate signatures on an ongoing basis. If logos are not recognized or remembered, they should be changed or dropped. If the provider's name is confusing, unimpressive, or too long, it should be changed to what communicates the intended information and impression to the intended audience. If the motto is unclear, not believed, or ignored, it should be modified or eliminated. If the motto truly expresses the provider's mission and values but is not believed, marketing must institute serious efforts in the areas of discovering, deciding, designing, and delivering.

Influencing Decisions

The ultimate purpose of describing, and of all marketing effort, is to influence the choices that persons make: reinforce and stimulate appropriate decisions or change inappropriate decisions. Essentially, marketing communications, together with other marketing efforts, can approach influencing decisions in two ways. First, it can discover what persons need, want, and wish for in making their choices and then design, deliver, and describe accordingly. This is a pure marketing approach, but probably impossible or inappropriate in its purest form for providers. Second, marketing can persuade persons to need, want, and wish for what they think they should, knowing that the sponsor offers precisely that. This is a pure sales approach and unlikely to be successful among assertive and independent consumers who have alternative choices, namely, competitors using a marketing approach.

In reality, a provider probably will need a combination of marketing and sales. People tend to think they have enough basic knowledge to choose the appropriate service and provider and to judge the quality of both, despite how much health care professionals might disagree. Given consumers' growing assertiveness with regard to health care choices and the growing number of competitors anxious to attract them, it is absolutely essential that physicians, nursing homes, and hospitals combine the ability to give people what they want with the ability to get them to want the right things.

Two basic approaches are available to influencing the criteria that persons use in making choices: education and sensitization. The *educational approach* describes what criteria people should use in judging services and providers, making a rational case for why those criteria are important. Such an approach must consciously strive not to be paternalistic and patronizing. Any attempt to convince the average citizen that the only important criteria are those used by professionals is sure to fail, and deservedly so. Consumers will rightly assert their insistence that their personal values be addressed in addition to professional standards.

The *sensitization approach* is indirect; it supplies information to consumers without trying to make a case that the information is essential to their choice. It relies, instead, on what is called the *agenda-setting effect* in communications.[3] By supplying information on a regular and attention-holding basis, providers can influence what customers think about, without necessarily changing what they believe. In effect, the purpose of sensitization is using repetition rather than argument to influence the criteria that people use in making judgments.

It is well established that in making most market decisions, consumers use at most a modest amount of information. In most choice situations, they initially think of or evoke to mind only one or two or perhaps three options. One study, for example, discovered that in 78 percent of nursing home choices, persons considered only one option.[4] Another study found that consumers considered an average of 2.6 criteria when choosing a breakfast cereal.[5] One may certainly speculate that people may tend to employ more information in selecting some providers, although no evidence suggests that they will consider dozens of criteria rather than a few. In my own research, the average number of reasons people have volunteered for choosing the last hospital they went to has been 3.1.

What complicates the choice process is that persons vary enormously in the options they call to mind (their evoked sets) and the criteria they use to choose among as many options as they call to mind (their attribute sets). A provider may use education and sensitization approaches to influence populations toward more uniform and fewer options, but only systematic discovery techniques can determine the provider's success. Since competing providers may be educating or sensitizing the same population differently, success in influencing large groups to employ the criteria that place one provider above another cannot be guaranteed.

A truism in conventional advertising states: "Never show them the factory!" This means that providers probably will only waste time describing the features they are proud of to audiences in the marketplace. Rather, the provider must be sure to talk about what interests the *audience*. Education may be used to influence what interests persons and sensitization may arouse new interests, but communications must address the audiences' interests, not the sponsor's. Discovery techniques should carefully monitor what criteria persons use in making their choices to ensure that education and sensitization and any other communication efforts are on target.

Timing of Messages

Another truism in advertising cites the most important factor in communication as "Repetition, Repetition, Repetition!" One certainly must regard communications effort as a permanent commitment rather than a one- or two-shot project. Even when an effective and efficient message, campaign, or strategy has had the desired effect, reinforcement is needed to maintain that effect against the erosion of time and the onslaughts of competitors. In general, a provider needs to repeat a specific message many times to ensure that the intended audience experienced it at least two or three times, the minimum number believed necessary for effect.

When the communications effort involves establishing a position in fresh minds, and especially changing a position in set minds, a substantial investment in high levels of exposure and repetition is probably required at the outset. Reinforcement and reminders require less but still need regular repetition. Only experience will reveal how many exposures over what period are needed for what effects with audiences. The audiences' present state of mind, the type of information to be communicated, and audiences' level of interest or involvement in the subject, as well as how well messages are designed and delivered will affect how many repetitions are needed. It is usually best to have too many rather than too few. Too few repetitions may produce no effect, suggesting that the entire effort was a waste of time, when in reality it might have come very close. Too many repetitions waste some resources but may at least show results; it takes quite a few too many before audiences become annoyed with repetitions and begin reversing the effect.

Guest Encounters

Health care providers should think of and use marketing communications as part of systematic building and maintaining of relationships, in addition to causing any specific desired effects. Communications should be planned so as to provide a permanent link with everyone with whom the provider wishes to establish and maintain a lasting relationship. With respect to individual patient care, communication contacts ideally should occur with each patient or family before, during, and after each care experience. Marketing communications should be used to attract guests and other customers, to promote satisfaction with specific care experiences, and to promote lasting relationships between the provider and its community.

Ongoing communications, including publicity, personal contact, word-of-mouth communications, media advertising, and direct delivery, should be used (1) to maintain awareness of the provider and its programs, (2) to supply information of interest to audiences, and (3) to reinforce each other. Newsletters, newspapers, feature stories, speakers' bureaus, regular ads, health advice columns, medical question and answer shows on radio or television are all ways to establish regular communication contacts. Comprehensive service programs, screening efforts, health fairs, and so on are also useful in promoting frequent personal contact to bolster the effects of communications.

Before individual care encounters, the provider should use communications to promote satisfaction and enhance the value of the encounter. Previsit or preadmission contacts can facilitate admission, promote confidence, explain care procedures, and answer any questions. Admission clerks who make the calls can make admitting appointments so that incoming patients will already know someone at the facility and feel expected when they arrive. Previsit contacts should be geared to establishing a personal relationship from the beginning between the organization and each guest.

Communications during encounters should enhance satisfaction and outcomes. Explanation of procedures to alleviate anxiety, assistance in the care process, expressions of concern and commitment, and advice on follow-up care are all examples of how communication can be used to increase satisfaction and thus subsequent use and positive word-of-mouth. Finding out each patient's expectations for each care encounter is the best way to start an effort aimed at satisfaction. Soliciting feedback throughout the care process is the best method to discover complaints while a chance exists to resolve them.

After each encounter, communications should be used to thank persons for choosing the provider, to gauge satisfaction, to reinforce follow-up care or advice, and to confirm the personal relationship between the provider and the guest. Such follow-up contacts should ideally be made by a person who cared for or at least visited the guest during the care experience, such as the primary nurse on the unit, a patient/resident visitor or representative, or a discharge planner. Admissions clerks may perform this task if they have established a personal relationship with patients. Ideally every patient will receive a follow-up contact, especially residents, inpatients, surgical outpatients and their families. Emergency room and clinic patients should also be contacted if feasible, at least on a sample basis. Increasingly, the provider should contact employers where worksite injuries, occupational health programs, or other customer relationships are involved.

Image vs. Product Communications

Much of the early effort in marketing communication by health care organizations was devoted to what would be termed *institutional advertising* in conventional marketing. It was devoted to self-praise, describing what a wonderful place X hospital, Y nursing home, or Z clinic was, typically employing vague claims on intangible dimensions. A favorite claim was likely to include something about "really caring" for patients, residents, or the entire community.

This approach has been widely ridiculed by advertising professionals, who have noted how competing institutions use exactly the same claims. Little evidence shows that such claims have succeeded in establishing or changing the public's perceptions of health care organizations. The current conventional wisdom espouses product advertising, which involves telling the public something specific and significant about individual services or packages of services, such as maternity, plastic surgery, and other definable "products." The contention is that people do not buy institutions, but rather specific categorical experiences relative to specific needs. Rather than describe the organization, marketers should describe what it sells.

Much of the logic behind these arguments is persuasive, under certain conditions. First, the purpose of communications is to reach people who do not have strong opinions about any organization and are interested in the specific services the organization has to sell. Second, the audiences for such messages will make or strongly influence the choice of provider. Third, the number of products the organization has to sell is manageable and the mix is compatible.

If persons already have strong loyalties to a specific organization, selling the virtues of a service offered by a competing organization will be difficult. For services such as maternity, plastic surgery, and alcohol treatment, where self-referral is common, product-specific communications make sense. For services that physicians dominate, however, advertising them to the public may anger the medical staff or referral sources, who think they should make the choice. As the number of services to be separately promoted increases, the cost of marketing communications efforts grows and the credibility of claims that one organization is the best one for many diverse services diminishes.

Given the importance of such intangible dimensions as continuity and confidence, both of which are easier to tie to an organization than a product, image-building or institutional advertising will probably still be used along with product-specific promotion. By focusing on the high-leverage customers as well as individual guests, the organization should be able to select the proper mix of the two approaches. By coordinating institutional and product-specific communication strategies, the organization can enhance the effects of both.

The marketing communications function is a major, permanent investment in any marketing effort. It is not anything that should be tried half-heartedly or tentatively, nor is it something that can be turned over to a marketing communications person or department. As with all marketing functions, it is too important to be left to marketers. Unless the organization embraces marketing communications and marketing itself as everybody's job, it is predetermining limited marketing success at best. Those providers that know they are delivering the best care owe it to themselves and to their communities to carry out the best marketing possible.

Footnotes

1. MacStravic, R.S. *Managing Health Care Marketing Communications.* Rockville, MD: Aspen Systems, 1986.

2. Inguanzo, J. and Harju, M. "How Do Consumers Receive Local Health Care Information?" *Hospitals* (April 1, 1985): 74.

3. McCombs, M. and Shaw, M. "The Agenda-Setting Effect of the Media." *Public Opinion Quarterly* 36 (1972): 49.

4. Froebe, D. et al. "Variables Influencing the Consumer's Choice of Nursing Homes." *Journal of Health Care Marketing* 2:2 (Spring 1982): 25.

5. Wright, P. "The Harrassed Decision Maker." *Journal of Applied Psychology* 59 (Oct. 1974): 555.

7.Evaluating

Evaluating efforts and results is as essential a component of the marketing function as it is of health care delivery. It involves two basic tasks: (1) determining what the effects of discovering, deciding, designing, delivery and describing efforts have been, then (2) deciding the value of such effects. The purpose of evaluation is primarily to learn how well each of the marketing tasks has been carried out and how much better each can be carried out in the future. Evaluation is not so much a separate step as it is a repetition of the marketing cycle: discovering what has and has not happened and deciding what has and has not worked, so that one can do a better job of designing, delivering, and describing next time.

Evaluating Discovery

Marketing can evaluate discovery efforts at two stages: before and after they are carried out. Before the fact, evaluation focuses on estimating if the value of the information to be gained from specific discovery efforts will be at least equal to the cost. After the fact, evaluation can compare actual value to actual cost and decide how discovery might have been more effective or efficient.

Any evaluation process must aim at accomplishing two separate tasks: (1) identifying what differences will be made (before the fact) or have been made (after the fact), then (2) determining what value those differences have to the organization. Evaluations before the fact are essentially the same as those made after an effort has been carried out, except that forecasts rather than measures of differences are used. The task of assigning a value to the forecast or measured differences is basically the same.

The value of discovery efforts comes from the intelligence, the relevant new knowledge, produced. The intelligence expected or gained from discovery should be evaluated in terms of its:

- *Validity and reliability:* Does it measure what it is supposed to (validity)? Would other valid approaches produce the same results (reliability)?
- *Accuracy and precision:* Is the information correct (accuracy)? Does it express findings within an appropriately narrow range of uncertainty (precision)?
- *Usefulness and actionability:* Can it be applied to what it was intended for so as to make a difference (usefulness)? Does a clear action response logically follow?
- *Timeliness:* Does it emerge in time to be used for its intended purpose?
- *Credibility:* Do the persons who are supposed to use the information have confidence in it? (Note that this may be affected by considerations beyond those of validity, reliability, accuracy, and precision.)

Before the fact, such considerations should be the basis on which discovery choices are made regarding the sample to be investigated, the information sought, questions used, sources examined, coding used, and scaling and analysis employed. After the fact, the marketer should seek independent confirmation by examining results obtained from a fresh perspective, ideally including a critical examination by someone not involved in the original planning. If one staff member or consultant develops the discovery approach, another should be used as evaluator, both before and after the approach is carried out. The second opinions should then be used as supplemental rather than superior guidance.

The value of intelligence gained through discovery may be determined through subjective discussions among those who are to use the results. This is often the simplest and most politically expedient approach. Marketing may employ specific group processes such as Delphi, nominal group, or focus group discussions to facilitate a group evaluation.[1] Problems with this approach emerge when the results have to be communicated and explained to others. Unless the participating group is a credible source of the intuitive judgments arrived at, a superior decision-making or reviewing body may not agree with its evaluation.

An alternative approach is to develop estimates of the choices or decisions that would have been made, the actions taken, and the results achieved, both with and without the intelligence gained from the discovery effort. Such estimates would still be developed through intuitive, subjective processes; the same group techniques would probably be used. Because objective estimates of the difference that the information will make or has made to the decision are made available, however, those who must review and agree with the value assigned can at least see what the value was based on.

For example, if several options were available and being considered before a discovery effort, marketing would examine those options against the different states of reality that might be found through discovery. The expected contribution to the provider's mission and vitality, if each option being considered were chosen and each possible state of reality were true, would then be estimated. Perhaps the choice involves a hospital's developing an immediate care center or not developing it. The states of reality possible might range from varying interest or opposition in the population served to apathy or enthusiasm among the medical staff. The probable results of such a decision under each relevant state of reality would likely vary from financial losses and medical staff revolt to profitability and stronger ties, with various intermediate possibilities.

Marketing would estimate the value to the hospital of having perfect knowledge in making such a choice compared to the potential costs of making choices without such knowledge. The value of perfect knowledge represents the upper bound of the potential value of any discovery effort. If the value of the potential difference made by having perfect information is not significantly greater than the cost of the discovery effort, then the effort should not be undertaken. Results of discovery efforts may always be as uncertain and unenlightening as present intuition. If the potential results are not much better than present intuition, considering the costs of obtaining them, then marketing should bypass the discovery step or develop a better approach.

It is helpful in evaluating the promise of a discovery effort to write a hypothetical report before undertaking it. This report should illustrate the types of intelligence expected and offer alternative answers to the questions addressed. If different answers to specific questions will not make any difference to possible decisions, then the questions probably should not be asked. If different results from the effort as a whole would make little or no difference to how the institution decides, designs, delivers, or describes, then the entire discovery effort may be pointless.

Evaluating Decisions

With or without discovery intelligence, marketing should evaluate the strategic and tactical decisions a provider makes in terms of con-tributions to its mission and vitality. Although other effects may be identifiable as results of decisions, the value of such effects should always by determined in terms of the organization's permanent values. Given the charitable missions of religious health care organizations, profitability is valued not only for its contribution to the organization's survival and vitality, but for its contribution to its ability to serve people from whom it will gain little or no revenue.

In religious health care, financial contributions from decisions represent important values, but these are instrumental rather than intrinsic. Positive bottom lines enable organizations to persevere and perhaps expand service to the community and the poor, in addition to providing capital for replacement and expansion. Every decision should be capable of having its expected and measured results assigned a value based on mission, even if the most direct and obvious results are financial. Any decision that has direct and obvious results related to mission will probably have other effects as well through its financial and organizational vitality impact.

Religious health care should probably alter its accounting reports to reflect this mission/vitality relationship. If service to the poor is its intent, the facility should separately show in its operational results how it has allocated the excess of revenue over expense to care of the poor. This care may take the form of discounted days of care and visits (for Medicaid and other partly paid patients) and free admissions, patient days, and treatments (for those unable to pay). These figures are more properly expressed as deliberate allocations from the bottom line rather than deductions from revenue. Although accounting principles may not support such a suggestion, this approach offers a clearer picture of how well a provider is carrying out its mission. It also shows how its marketing success in attracting and satisfying paying patients enables it to maintain its charitable mission.

For effective evaluation of decisions, as well as of design, delivery, and description, the provider must have a clear statement of mission and a clearly identified set of value commitments. The organization should be able to measure the state of such values before and after making and implementing a decision; this provides a basis for evaluating the decision. If the provider has commitments to community service, it should be able to measure whether it has expanded, contracted, or maintained its service to the community as a result of a decision. If it has commitments to system leadership; technical quality; patient, employee, and physician satisfaction; operational productivity and efficiency; community trust; health status; or any other valued parameter, it should be regularly monitoring what is happening to each.

The value of a decision comes from its total impact on the organization's set of values as well as on the intended outcomes. Side effects, both positive and negative, contribute to the worth of a decision and should be considered before and examined after the fact. How all organizational values have been affected—whether protected, enhanced, or damaged by a decision—determines whether it was a good one.

In a marketing effort, a decision's value begins with the impact it has on the provider's market position. Impact should always be gauged first in terms of market size and market share. The objectives of any marketing decision, whether strategic or tactical, should be stated in terms of maintained, increased, or decreased market (e.g., total utilization of a type of service; enrollment in HMOs, PPAs, CMPs, or employer contracts) and the share of that market achieved, increased, decreased, or maintained by the organization and its particular programs.

The market objectives and results affect organizational values first in the utilization and revenue effects they produce, then in the mission and vitality contributions attributable to such effects. When marketing is applied to employee and physician recruitment or retention, similar operational effects would come first, such as numbers of employees or physicians, absenteeism, turnover, percentage of physician admissions, and referrals. These would then be linked to mission or vitality measures as appropriate.

The provider should not rely on operational measures as direct indicators of marketing decision effects. Overall health care use might increase or decrease regardless of a marketing decision, or it might change in a way that would lead to the wrong conclusion about effects. For example, use of a given program might decrease because total use of that service in the market has decreased. In such a case, the provider's share of the market rather than its level of utilization will indicate whether its efforts have had beneficial results. In the same way, use of a program might increase because of an overall rise in the market, perhaps from a flu epidemic or extreme weather conditions. Under such circumstances, use of a provider's services might increase substantially, but not as a result of its marketing effort.

In general, all health service marketing efforts should have demonstrable impact on overall use of a given service and/or the provider's share of that use. In some cases, efforts aim at the timing rather than amount of use, such as earlier detection or less fluctuation. Decisions in both planning and evaluation should focus first on market measures in looking for effect, then on operational measures and organizational values in assigning worth to any effect.

Evaluating Design

Marketing should evaluate the value of design efforts, both before and after their implementation primarily in terms of the resulting attractiveness to prospects. A management perspective also requires that such concerns as operational feasibility, effects on technical quality, productivity and efficiency, and revenues and expenditures be considered as well. In most cases, design effects can be gauged in comparison to marketing and operational performance before implementation of design changes. When a new program is involved, however, marketing must gauge design effects against estimated performance based on the alternatives rejected.

As with decision efforts, design efforts should aim at specific, measurable objectives. Whereas decisions are judged in terms of market measures, designs are judged according to specific preference measures. When design aims at increasing the attractiveness of an existing program through specific modifications to benefits (product), access (place), or costs (price), it should be able to anticipate impact by surveying the market to see how the new design will affect stated preference and intentions. After the fact, design depends for effect on delivery, if satisfaction is concerned, and on description, if attraction is concerned.

The specific focus of design efforts is on the evoked set placement of the provider or its programs in the minds of intended markets. Design should be judged by how many people rate the provider or program their best choice or only acceptable choice vs. how many place it lower. These measures of preference are the intended areas of effect. The value of design effects are then a function of the market measures, operational measures, and mission and vitality values that can be traced or otherwise attributed to preference effects.

Given the variability and unpredictability of the link between preference and use, a delay or difference may occur between the two. Achieving a high preference for a new maternity program may not be followed by any utilization impact for nine months or more, since women are reluctant to change providers in the middle of pregnancy. Achieving a high preference among younger persons may produce a low impact on use of inpatient care because younger persons use less care. At most, design can be held accountable for reinforcement of or shifts in preference, together with the promise of whatever management improvements are anticipated. Changes in market size or share, in use, and in revenues and mission contributions will ideally follow, but these depend on other efforts as well.

Evaluating Delivery

The principal focus of delivery efforts is on guest or customer satisfaction, although delivery has an indirect impact on attraction through description efforts. Marketing should evaluate specific delivery steps in terms of both specific guest ratings and overall satisfaction. Moreover, probes of specific dimensional ratings (competence, caring, convenience, etc.) should produce at least some indication that specific delivery innovations were the reasons for improvements in ratings. Since the effects of delivery innovations are often unpredictable and diffuse, a less than perfect correlation will exist between specific changes in setting, props, characters, costumes, action, or dialogue and the intended judgment dimension. Probing will add to understanding of guests' interpretation of specific changes, even if it finds unexpected impacts.

Using ongoing, systematic guest satisfaction monitoring, providers can evaluate delivery innovations throughout the year as each is implemented. This provides the rationale for using a flexible satisfaction monitoring approach, which can be changed as often as significant delivery innovations are implemented. Providers should also examine community preference surveys for indirect effects of delivery innovations, although description efforts may also be involved in any effects detected.

The value of delivery effects is far more difficult to gauge than are the effects themselves. Individual judgment dimension ratings should be linked to overall satisfaction in some demonstrable fashion; however, satisfaction does not have even as clear a connection to market measures, operational measures, and organizational values as does community preference. Changing evoked set preference positions of the provider should be closely but imperfectly linked to changes in market shares. Achieving high satisfaction among current guests or increasing satisfaction levels may prevent the loss of volume and encourage subsequent use of services, but this is much more difficult to tie to measurable market effects than changes in attraction and preference ratings.

On the other hand, satisfaction of patients has a legitimate claim as an intrinsic value. High satisfaction tends to lead to greater compliance, fewer broken appointments, better care results, fewer malpractice suits, and better patient payment, as well as enhanced quality of life for patients, employees, and physicians. In many ways, the marketing benefits of enhanced satisfaction, although difficult to gauge, are serendipitous side effects to their other known, but also difficult to measure, benefits.

Evaluating Description

The effects of description efforts are perhaps the easiest to identify but can be the most difficult to place a value on. Description aims at placing or keeping the provider or its programs in positions as best known options or establishing specific knowledge or attitudes in the minds of the public. The effects of description should be detectable through community and guest surveys in terms of such factors as whether and how many persons:

- Have been exposed to a given message, and how many times
- Recall or recognize specific messages and their content
- Are aware of specific information about the provider and its programs
- Associate positive subjective judgments and feelings with the provider and its programs
- Intend to behave in some specific desired fashion

Traditional advertising evaluations tend to focus on measures of exposure, repetition, recall, and recognition. Although these are easy and inexpensive to measure, they are essentially useless as bases for assigning value. They are strong on the side of detecting effect but outrageously weak on the side of assigning value to the effects. Numbers of persons exposed, repetitions, and whether persons recall or recognize messages are not signs that they have changed or added to knowledge, beliefs, attitudes, and intentions in their minds. Even states of mind are difficult to tie with any degree of certainty to market or operational objectives and thus to mission or vitality values.

It is helpful and perhaps even necessary to monitor exposures, repetitions, recall, and recognition to trace any effects on persons' minds to their causes. It is these effects rather than the causes, however, that represent value to the provider. Evaluation of description efforts should almost always be done internally or by consultants not associated with those responsible for developing and implementing marketing communications strategies, campaigns, and messages. Moreover, evaluation should look for specific evidence of knowledge, beliefs, attitudes, and intentions that can be attributed to communications effort. Asking new patients where they heard about a given program or how they learned about the provider should be a routine part of the admissions and intake process, at least on a sample basis.

Relationship Evaluation

Although providers should evaluate each of the marketing tasks separately and systematically, the relationships between the organization and its critical publics (patients, community, physicians, its employees, area employers, volunteers, donors, etc.) properly represent the chief focus of evaluation. Individual evaluation efforts should focus on the effects expected from specific discovery, decision, design, delivery, and description investments. In the long run, however, it is the number of persons with whom the provider has been able to achieve and sustain the intended relationships that shows how effective overall marketing efforts have been.

The provider needs to identify both the people and the organizations that form the markets and segments with whom it wishes to have lasting relationships. It should identify as clearly and measurably as possible the nature of such relationships. Then it should systematically monitor the status of such relationships and the tangible as well as intangible bases for them. The provider should systematically manage critical relationships, using the same marketing principles and techniques traditionally associated with marketing specific services.

Relationship marketing strives to achieve a special place in persons' minds: whenever they feel the need for a health service similar to the one the organization offers, persons will think of and contact the organization (or one of its physicians) more or less automatically. To achieve such a position requires that the organization develop appropriate responses to almost every possible need that a given population would perceive. The most obvious populations are those who share a life status and set of health needs that distinguish them from other populations and bind them together; that is, persons who form a true market segment. Examples include women (working, pregnant), the elderly (frail, hearty, somewhat dependent), the chronically ill (diabetic persons, hypertensive persons), and fitness enthusiasts.

Conventional marketing strategies would suggest looking for specific opportunities throughout the market or following a brand extension approach. *Brand extension,* or product line marketing, starts with a specific type of service and seeks to extend the range of the service in any direction available. A cancer treatment service, for example, would search for ways to go backward to prevention and early detection, then forward to rehabilitation and hospice care. A market extension or relationship management approach starts with a population and consciously aims at providing, managing, or at least sponsoring a network that will respond to every probable health need of that population.

Such a strategy requires deliberately extending the provider's vision beyond conventional medical models of care. It may mean opening up possibilities of incorporating acupuncturists, podiatrists, chiropractors, and massage therapists in addition to orthopedists in a sports and fitness relationship effort. Maternity relationship programs might include nurse midwives and family practitioners in addition to obstetricians and labor-delivery-recovery and outpatient delivery in addition to conventional services. Nursing home programs could be extended to include home health services, outpatient physical therapy, and so forth to become a comprehensive resource for the elderly.

Evaluating a relationship, especially one intended to be lasting and personal, requires a special effort. In addition to systematic patient satisfaction monitoring and regular community surveys, the knowledge, attitudes, and behavior of past patients should be separately surveyed. Specific market segments, such as pregnant or working women, elderly persons, and diabetic patients, should be contacted to learn if the desired relationship has been established and if it is satisfying.

Marketers would ask members of any market or segment selected questions regarding their:

- Awareness of the range of services offered by the provider
- Knowledge of how to obtain needed services
- Preferred responses to specific problems or needs
- Feelings about recent care experiences
- Overall attitude toward the organization
- Recall of and attitudes toward the organization's communications
- Perceived and unsolved problems and needs

In effect, relationship marketing and management require their own set of discovery, decision, design, delivery, and description efforts, all aimed at establishing and maintaining the intended lasting relationship with selected markets and segments. The approaches used by a hospital should serve as a model for the relationship marketing and management efforts of its medical staff. The hospital can then use its evaluation efforts to simultaneously monitor awareness, knowledge, attitudes, and behavior regarding its medical staff members. The hospital can pass on its experience and expertise in relationship marketing and management to the medical staff in order to improve the effectiveness of their efforts. By improving the practice development success of medical staff members, the hospital improves its own professional relations and marketing success as well.

Maintaining satisfactory and lasting relationships with entire markets and sets of patients as well as with the medical staff has powerful and immediate benefit to any marketing efforts by hospitals. As the system moves toward macromarketing in addition to micromarketing, the benefits increase.[2] As employers, insurance organizations, government, and other buyers increase their involvement in the selective purchasing of health care, the ability to offer comprehensive packages of services and manage relationships with entire populations will become not only advantageous but necessary. The hospital that can manage the health of entire populations and the cost, quality, and access of services for those populations will have a significant if not overwhelming market advantage.

The hospital looking forward will already be designing if not operating the kind of marketing, management, and information systems needed for success in population relationship micromarketing as well as macromarketing. Evaluation of macromarketing efforts include monitoring of the health status and health service expenditures of populations together with their knowledge and attitudes toward the hospital. As financing of health care systems moves toward capitation contracting, the hospitals that can offer proven comprehensive health service packages and satisfying relationships will prosper. Those that cannot will disappear or be absorbed up by those that can.

Nursing homes should work toward developing comprehensive systems to serve their basic markets of the frail elderly. Home health care, congregate care, and even retirement housing projects can serve as feeder mechanisms for new residents as well as additional sources of revenue. Networking with other providers, including hospitals and physicians, can help maintain awareness levels and keep the nursing home as first choice among, for example, discharge planners. Moreover, such systems can take advantage of economies of scale, shared services, and comprehensive medical records to improve efficiency and quality.

Footnotes

1. Delbecq, A. et al. *Group Techniques for Program Planning*. Glenview, IL: Scott, Foresman, 1975.

2. MacStravic, R.S. "Macro-Marketing in Health Care." *Hospital & Health Services Administration* 30:3 (May/June 1983).

8. Values and Marketing Evidence

Many persons have attempted to describe how religious health care could or should be different from commercial business, for-profit, or even non-religious health care. Most discuss the manifestation of religious values in relations with employees, physicians, patients, family members, and the general public. Since this is a marketing discussion, it will focus on outward and visible signs of religious values as they affect relations with customers, and attempts to maintain or improve the attraction and satisfaction of guests.

From a marketing perspective, it is useful to view the manifestation of religious values as a process of discovering, deciding, designing, delivering, and describing evidence of such values in ways that will contribute to the achievement of marketing goals. What religious commitments call on health professionals to do often overlaps or fits well with what customers want them to do. This applies more to a health care situation than any other.

Religious values do not necessarily conform to marketing logic at the strategic level. A businesslike marketing approach is unlikely to produce a special commitment to the poor and powerless unless good profits can be made there. Marketing has no values of its own; however, users can employ it as a tool in furthering any set of values they select. The religious provider can use marketing strategies and techniques to attract more poor and powerless persons if its commitments demand and its survival permits this.

Commitments to individual dignity and worth, to the equality of all persons, to personal growth; participatory decision making; and similar expressions of religious values are likely to promote good employee and community relations. The basis for such commitments may not be their practical management effects, but they probably will promote organizational success if implemented.

Religious values expressed in dealings with patients and families are totally consistent with marketing. Consider the commitments that religious values typically involve:

- Respect for individual dignity and worth
- Concern for others, commitments to service
- Beliefs in the sharing of power and responsibility
- Concern for social, psychological, and spiritual health
- Beliefs in honesty and openness in communication
- Commitments to social justice and to fair dealings

These values call on members of religious health care organizations to devote their efforts toward living out such commitments in their day-to-day relations with patients and families. Mission effectiveness programs are used to monitor and enhance the extent to which such values are manifested. Retreats, informal and formal discussions, and other forms of self-assessment help maintain the organization's focus on its basic religious values and avoid tendencies to focus on more easily measured business realities.

Self-assessment efforts are a legitimate and necessary approach to maintaining a focus on religious values and commitments. They can be usefully supplemented by a second approach: religious health care providers can ask their patients, co-workers, and others, "How well are we doing from your point of view?" Whether they are more likely to be right in their assessment is unimportant. On the other hand, if others find these providers' behavior inconsistent with or irrelevent to their espoused values, those asking this question should at least reflect on the answers.

Marketing insists that health professionals look at everything from the customer's perspective. The ancient maxim that the customer is always right does not subjugate judgment to customers; it merely recognizes the reality that what customers perceive is true to them and drives their behavior in the market. Whenever a service organization claims to be providing good or even excellent service, the marketing professional will insist that customers be polled to determine how they see it. The customers may not be correct in any abstract sense, but what they perceive is what counts from a marketing perspective.

This same logic applies to the question of how well health personnel are living out their espoused values. If they are committed to respecting the individual dignity and worth of everyone they relate to, they should probably ask at least a sample of these others whether they sense such respect. If health care workers fail to express their commitments in ways that are clear to others, they are missing an opportunity for testimony. They are also likely to be missing a chance to enhance their relations with customers.

Discovering

Religious health care providers can ask patients, family members, and the general public many questions to discover how well they are expressing their values:
- Do they find staff members (physicians, employees) caring, compassionate, sensitive, and concerned?
- Do they feel that staff members show respect, courtesy, and friendliness and treat them as special persons?
- Do they feel that staff members identified and responded to their total needs?
- How do they rate staff members on honesty, openness, trust, informativeness, and understandability of communication?
- Do they feel they were equal participants in the care process, in making decisions regarding care?
- How do they rate staff members on their helpfulness, attentiveness, and thoroughness?
- Do patients and families understand the care processes, diagnoses, prognoses, and implications of their illnesses?
- To what extent do patients and families sense a loving environment, cheerful gentleness, comforting reassurance, and reverential regard?

Marketing would then go one step further:
- What evidence did people use in arriving at their conclusions?
- What, in their minds, were the signals of caring and compassion, of concern and respect?
- What conveyed gentleness and sensitivity to them?
- In what ways did staff members demonstrate a reverent courtesy, cheerfulness, and helpfulness?

Discovering the evidence that persons rely on in assessing behavior gives health care workers the information they need to furnish proof of their commitments. It also provides a basis for promoting good patient, family, and public relations from a marketing perspective. This evidence, especially those tangible signals that are mentioned by many persons, can then be designed into (or out of) the patient experience, delivered on a day-to-day basis as demonstrations of the organization's values, and described in its marketing communications.

Deciding

Information gained through probing patient and family perceptions will provide the basis for determining what specific patterns of behavior might be initiated, eliminated, or modified in the interest of better demonstrating organizational values. The number of people mentioning specific behaviors will suggest the impact potential of any change. The costs, feasibility, and side effects of any specific idea will have to be considered together with its positive effects.

If discovery efforts work well, the information will readily translate into management decisions. For example, patients might be asked to rate the staff on their caring, compassion, or concern. Following the rating question, a probing question might be: "What did (the staff) do that best showed how (caring, concerned, compassionate) they are?" Another probe might ask: "In what way(s) did (staff) express their (caring, concern)?"

The more specific the probing questions are, the more tangible, specific, and manageable will be the responses. The challenge in deciding will be to select the behaviors that will be both effective and efficient in demonstrating the traits that patients want and that the organization is committed to showing. Health organizations often shout about how caring they are, sometimes as much as how excellent they are in quality of care. The organizations that can determine what evidence of caring and excellence they can deliver most effectively and efficiently will gain significant marketing advantage.

Delivering

In most cases, the identification of significant evidence, when published to staff members, will motivate appropriate responses. When physicians, nurses, and other caregivers learn that taking time with patients, gentle touching, or some other action is among the most frequently mentioned signals of caring, they are likely to respond accordingly. The specific patterns of behavior suggested by patients as the best evidence of desirable traits should be supplemented by the ideas of staff members. Marketing circles will develop their own forms of evidence based on the insights and experience of staff members. Patient feedback will confirm how well such evidence works.

In addition to the motivational power of patient-suggested evidence, management can promote innovations in staff behavior by testing out specific ideas on a small scale. One nursing unit might adopt a type of evidence suggested by patients or staff members and monitor patient comments to check results. If patient feedback continues to include examples of evidence in response to probing questions, it will indicate how well specific initiatives work in two ways. First, it will show whether patient ratings of specific traits (caring, helpfulness, responsiveness to complete needs, etc.) have improved, declined, or stayed the same. Second, the pattern of answers to probing questions will show whether patients and family members noticed the evidence supplied.

Depending on the type of evidence cited by patient feedback or suggested by staff members, management may promote initiatives or simply support staff efforts. If initiatives can be implemented by staff without management involvement, staff members gain both speed and enthusiasm. If management is needed, the fact that initiatives originated with patients or staff will facilitate implementation in most cases. In addition, staff morale should improve and the organization will broaden its commitments to its employees.

This basic approach of searching for the evidence can be used with physicians and employees as well as with patients, families, and communities. Physicians and employees are in many ways the customers of the organization. They have choices, and how they made those choices can affect the mission and survival success of the organization. How they perceive the organization, its administration, and its management will greatly influence how they make their choices. Once the organization knows which evidence means what to physicians and employees, it is also in a better position to manage its relations with these vital customers.

Description

The use of evidence may have its greatest value in the description function of marketing. Assuming that the religious health care organization wishes to be seen as caring, compassionate, courteous, helpful, responsive to the totality of patient needs, and so forth, it can best promote its reputation in the community if it knows and talks about those facts that communicate positive attributes to others. Any organization can claim to be caring, helpful, informative, honest, and respectful, but how many can prove it?

The key to successful use of evidence in marketing communication is first to use the right evidence. It is equally important for the organization to make sure that the evidence communicated is delivered in fact as well as described in words, sounds, or pictures. Failing to deliver what is described, especially when it is objective, tangible evidence rather than fuzzy, puffy generalizations, is sure to promote dissatisfaction. This in turn will promote negative word-of-mouth communication, which will both counter the organization's marketing communication and undermine public trust in everything it says.

Examples of Evidence

Very little published literature discusses what types of evidence demonstrate specific positive attributes in the minds of patients, family members, and the general public. Moreover, persons are likely to vary in their interpretation of specific items of evidence. Proven forms of evidence that will invariably communicate a given trait to all persons in all situations are unlikely to exist. This makes it all the more important for each organization to do its own discovering.

To illustrate the sorts of specifics that might be cited as evidence for particular traits, a study of a rural community's attitudes toward physicians cited the following behaviors:

- *Evidence of caring*—spending time with patients, avoiding the appearance of being rushed; knowing and using persons' names, family backgrounds, and previous encounters; asking about concerns beyond the specific problem that motivated the visit; following up each visit with a phone call to check on progress
- *Evidence of honesty and trust*—being thorough and open in discussing the diagnosis, prognosis, therapy, and causes of problems; using understandable language; asking if patients have any questions and answering them
- *Evidence of competence and skill*—being thorough in examination and interviewing; reaching a confident diagnosis quickly yet openly admitting uncertainty and being willing to call in assistance; knowing the patient's previous history and family situation (Note: Experience indicates that physician appearance, mode of dress, diplomas and certificates, and other nonbehavioral items are also evidence of competence.)

These findings indicate that the same evidence signal more than one positive trait. Taking time with patients and being thorough in examination and explanation are signs of caring, trustworthiness, and competence. Demonstrating knowledge of the patient's background is a sign of both competence and caring. Using understandable language was cited as evidence of honesty, but also of competence and informativeness. Rarely did more than a third of the respondents mention the same item of evidence for a given trait, but most cited each of four or five items as evidence of one of the positive traits examined.

One may argue that consciously managing behavior to provide evidence of positive traits is a way of misleading the public. This could be true if uncaring, dishonest, and incompetent care providers adopt the trappings of such traits without the substance. On the other hand, if the caring, honest, and competent care providers cannot demonstrate those qualities to the public and patients, they may be depriving many of their superior talents and leaving the field to those who are simply clever at marketing.

Communicating Evidence

Evidence may be used with communications aimed at asserting a specific positive trait. To back up a claim of caring, for example, providers could cite the amount of time spent with patients or the follow-up efforts they make. To support claims regarding honesty and trust, providers could promise to use understandable language, to answer questions, and discuss concerns in full. As evidence of competence, providers might promise to spend time with patients until they fully understand their problems and the choices available to them.

Since many effects may characterize specific items of evidence, many might be used without any mention of a positive trait. A hospital might point to its nurses giving back rubs, tucking in patients at night, and taking personal responsibility for only a few patients at a time as evidence of caring, but the hospital knows that many will see these as signs of competence, trust, helpfulness, and perhaps many other traits as well. When specific, objective behavior patterns are communicated, their factual, verifiable nature will make them far more believable than an unsubstantiated claim.

Testimonials are a popular and effective way to communicate positive traits. Having a former patient describe the caring, competent, and attentive nurses; the attractive and comfortable building; and the tasty food and convenient parking is likely to prove more effective than having a paid spokesperson do the same. Including evidence in the testimonial can supplement the effect in two ways. First, it can make the testimonial more credible by showing that it was based on hard evidence. Second, including the hard evidence can promote perceptions of other positive traits that the testifier does not mention.

With the help of evidence, all types of positive traits can be more effectively communicated than with claims or even testimonials alone. Of particular importance in marketing religious health care are those traits that correspond to the values and commitments of the sponsoring religious institute. All such values relate to the way care providers will behave with respect to patients. No reason exists for religious health care to be more competent, convenient, reasonably priced, or otherwise superior in impersonal terms. Some very good reasons exist, however, for why it might be more caring, trustworthy, complete, and otherwise personally satisfying.

The dynamics of marketing challenge religious health care to translate its lofty rhetoric into tangible evidence that will demonstrate its virtues to the people it serves. The best place to start is learning what evidence people use in making judgments about care providers, especially those judgments reflecting the values and commitments intrinsic to the sponsoring community or organization. If superior forms of evidence exist, providers are justified in using them for their own self-assessments. It might also be worth the effort to educate the public toward use of more appropriate evidence.

As Tom Peters has pointed out, the general public makes judgments about important traits on the basis of the evidence that is available and that means something to them.[1] The airline traveler may interpret the coffee stain on a tray as a sign of poor engine maintenance. Pilots and others more familiar with airline operation might laugh at such an interpretation. If providers cannot supply better evidence, however, they would be foolish to remain satisfied with the negative, inaccurate conclusions that customers reach. If providers deserve to be judged in positive terms by those they serve, they should not leave their judgments to chance.

Effects of Evidence

The principal effect of evidence in health care marketing is to promote attraction of additional patients and other customers by increasing the credibility and effect of communications. If the correct types of evidence have been identified in the discovery process, and are used correctly in the description process, more persons should be persuaded regarding the superior health care experience offered. The experience that is superior in terms of what patients want as well as what providers view as important warrants increased volume.

A second and equally important effect of evidence is in promoting satisfaction and attraction. A provider that focuses on its caring, complete, helpful, informative, loving, and respectful employees risks that its patients will expect to find proof of such traits but may fail to do so. Unless the provider's ideas of evidence are consistent with how patients arrive at their judgments, each claimed trait may arouse expectations that will not be fulfilled. By contrast, describing specific evidence will tend to focus expectations toward that evidence, enabling the provider to deliver exactly what was described. The communicated evidence can persuade prospective patients that the provider possesses desirable traits, and the delivered experience will prove it.

Specifying evidence in marketing communications can also have a third valuable effect. This involves publically announcing objective realities that should be characteristic of patient experience, which should promote the staff's adherence to such announcements. Each employee and physician might have different ideas about what traits such as caring mean and therefore about what each is expected to do. Specifying the objective evidence of caring that means the most to patients calls on each physician and employee to spend the time, know the background, and live up to such patient expectations.

Moreover, translating positive traits or attributes into tangible evidence should promote provider and employee morale. Those seriously committed to be caring, honest, helpful, and sensitive might find it difficult to determine if they are reflecting these traits as they should or could be. By translating such commitments into observable behavior that is significant to patients, caregivers themselves can monitor their performance and promote positive feedback from patients.

Marketing and Values

Marketing is a pragmatic discipline. It employs an understanding of market dynamics and human behavior in an engineering process designed to bring about benefits to those who employ it well. Marketing is a tool capable of being used for many purposes, some admirable and some not. Because it is based on the necessity of promising and delivering what people want, marketing has potential for doing much good, as well as also causing much harm. People want many things that will harm them in the long run and do not always want what will do them the most good. A natural limit is imposed on how much harm can be done, since even the cleverest marketer cannot fool all the people all the time.

The great potential for good inherent in marketing lies in its ability to respond to what people want with what really is good for them. Combining professionally excellent health care with what patients define as excellence results in superior care. It is a foolhardy and self-defeating conceit to be content with offering excellent care and blaming the uninformed and misguided public for looking elsewhere. If providers are as good as the values they espouse, they should make certain they are good enough in the eyes of the public to survive and succeed in their mission.

An arguable position states that religious health care enjoys a significant potential marketing advantage. To the health care business, motivated by profit, service is a means rather than an end. As a means, service excellence will be pursued as far as is necessary to achieve profit goals, and no farther. By contrast, religious health care is committed to excellence in service as an end, with successful financial outcomes as a means to that end. This means that excellence in service should be pursued as far as it can be, constrained only by the financial necessity. Those who pursue excellence in service as an end should find themselves ahead of those who deal with it only as means.

Translating this into evidential terms, religious health care should be pursuing behavior that will demonstrate its values and should take that behavior as far as possible. Physicians and employees who share such commitments should be constantly looking for ways to be more caring, concerned, honest, helpful, responsive, and reassuring. Those who regard health care merely as a business will look for ways to be as caring, concerned, helpful, honest, responsive, and reassuring as they have to be. Religious health care organizations should always be ahead, forcing others to try and catch up.

The use of evidence offers a way to be more effective in marketing and more excellent in service at the same time. What health care customers want from health care at least includes the same values and commitments that religious health care espouses. The motivation for being respectful of human dignity and worth, concerned for the total well-being of all, and promotive of understanding and justice is not to achieve marketing success. For this reason, because marketing is a means rather than an end, religious health care should be better at using it.

Footnotes

1. Peters, T. "Common Courtesy: The Ultimate Barrier to Entry." *Hospital Forum* (Jan./Feb. 1984): 10.

9. Marketing Stragety

A place exists in people's minds that religious health care organizations can aspire to: their personal provider in contrast to more bureaucratic, impersonal businesses that offer similar services. Not everyone in a population may be interested in having a personal hospital or nursing home in the same sense that they have a personal physician. After all, anywhere from 15 to 25 percent of any population probably does not have a personal physician. On the other hand, significant potential advantages accompany achieving and maintaining a position in the minds of many people as their personal provider.

Other service organizations, such as banks, have become less personal over time. They use machines instead of people to serve customers. They have high turnover in tellers, so that even old and regular customers are strangers and often are treated as such. Many banks offer a special service to their large depositors, including separate entrances and VIP treatment, but have lost their places as personal institutions for the masses.

As health care organizations increasingly adopt business practices and ways of thinking, they are likely to lose their claims on people's minds as personal providers. Cutting back on unprofitable services and pushing for lower costs to increase profit will tend to undermine trust. Commitment to service can coexist with desire for profit, but when profit becomes the end and service the means, that is likely to show in the ways people are treated.

Importance of Personal Traits

Most of the subjective judgment factors that persons rely on in choosing and judging health care providers are personal attributes. An institution can be convenient, can have reasonable costs, can be comfortable, and can offer choices to its customers. Competence, caring, continuity, confidence, courtesy, commitment, and communicativeness, however, are characteristics of persons, not places or products. Persons may attribute such characteristics to institutions, but only through association with staff members at such institutions.

Any design or delivery approach to improving or maintaining the organization's reputation on intangible judgment factors will necessitate focusing on how persons in the organization look, act, and communicate. Administration may alter the organization's reputation for comfort, convenience, cost, and control by making some dramatic change in furnishings or temperature, in locations or hours, in charges, or in choices offered to patients. Even these relatively tangible dimensions are affected by personal interactions between patients and physicians or employees. The intangible dimensions, although susceptible to administrative effort in the form of policy, procedure, and leadership, are essentially characteristics that can only be associated with institutions if they are demonstrated by persons who are part of those institutions.

Competence, for example, is something that people have and demonstrate, even though machines may have something close in terms of state-of-the-art technology. To have faith in the competence of an organization, it is necessary to believe in the competence of its people. Continuity is almost totally a personal factor; it comes from seeing familiar faces and being recognized and greeted by providers and other employees as an old friend. This can be enhanced by good record keeping so that members of the organization can remind themselves about established patients and their family, work, and social backgrounds. Continuity, however, is demonstrated and communicated by people.

Caring is a uniquely personal trait. One can talk about a caring institution, but only persons can care. Commitment is equally restricted to personal attitudes, even though one could make a list of organizational commitments. Only persons can credibly demonstrate a sense of caring and commitment. Confidence is something a person has in others, although a sense of trust can be established relative to an institution. Confidence in an organization, however, denotes trust in its traditions and values, as demonstrated by its members' behavior. Trust comes from what persons say and do. Patients trust an organization when they believe in its members.

Only people can deliver courtesy; machines may be efficient and accurate, even comfortable and convenient, but never courteous. Respect is also reserved as a human trait. Although communicativeness may involve technologies such as telephones and computers, it relies essentially on people. Only people can be sensitive to what patients, residents, and family members want to know and whether they understood what was said. Even control or choice factors require the participation of people to communicate and arrange options, although making them available is an organizational act.

Partnership and Personalization

Among the more powerful developments in the health care marketplace is the growing desire among many for a true *partnership* in the care process. Patients are asking for significant roles in health care decisions. Family members of nursing home residents are reacting favorably to programs that offer them a continuing, significant role in the care of their loved one. Partnerships are personal relationships. Someone can feel like a partner of a place or thing, but it is easier to feel like a partner of a person.

Many situations exist in which being a religious health care organization carries an automatic market advantage. If many persons in the service population espouse the same religion and feel more comfortable in, have greater confidence in, or otherwise prefer institutions sponsored by their religion, the advantage can be significant. In such circumstances, it is also likely that significant numbers of persons may deliberately seek care elsewhere because they are not of the same religion as the institution.

Many situations also occur in which the particular religion is of little advantage, because of relatively few persons in the area who espouse that religion. In such circumstances, the particular religion is also less likely to be a disadvantage. The key, however, is to make the fact that it is a *religious* health care organization, an important and positive factor in the minds of those choosing and judging competing alternatives. This may best be accomplished through personalizing the organization. Religious health care organizations have a greater potential for such personalization.

Religions share traditions that focus on people. Beginning with a personal God, religions also have personal heroes, or individuals that have so exemplified the religion's values that they are revered and referred to constantly. Religious health care organizations have heroes as well. Stories about their founders and other persons associated with the organization's development and operation are important components of their traditions. In contrast to for-profit organizations, for example, religious health care organizations are guided by congregations or religious institutes, that is, groups of people, rather than by corporations.

The challenge in personalizing the organization is to think, act, and communicate the answer to the question: *"Who* are we?" rather than

"What are we?" Effectively answering this question in decision, design, and delivery and then in description stages of marketing can produce a competitive advantage to overcome what may be the business disadvantages of being a religious health care organization.

Religious health care organizations seem to share commitments that are not always in the best short-range business tradition. Commitments to the dignity and worth of every individual impose some requirements and limitations that may interfere with short-run productivity, efficiency, and profit. Commitments to the needs of the whole person, including psychosocial and spiritual as well as medical needs, may require a wider range of responses that add to costs without adding to revenue. Commitments to disadvantaged persons may reduce revenues and add to costs.

In the long run at least, religious providers can hope that such commitments will promote rather than threaten their survival in a competitive marketplace and in the community. Prospective and present customers may find a religious health care organization more attractive and satisfying because of its commitments. Communities may find them more deserving of support, including financial and legal assistance. The challenge is to live out and communicate the organization's internal values in such a way as to demonstrate its value to customers and community. The personal provider organization is a promising basis for doing so.

Internal Marketing Steps

To become known as the personal health care provider organization first requires marketing to develop design and delivery steps that personalize the service experience. This should begin with internal marketing strategies that encourage employees to feel that they *are* the organization rather than its servants. Having employees represented on the governing board or on permanent advisory bodies are among the ways of promoting this attitude through formal structural steps. Just as hospitals are promoting the concept of partnership with their medical staffs, all health care organizations should promote a sense that their employees are in all but a fiduciary sense *owners* of the service business.

The organization's heroes should be constantly cited as personal embodiments of the values and personality of the organization. Those heroes still alive, even if retired, should be encouraged to communicate the organization's personality by their presence, words, and actions. Those heroes that belong to the organization's past should be made familiar through both formal and informal communication. Both stirring heroic acts and personal anecdotes about founders, prior administrators, managers, employees, volunteers, and board members should be as familiar to new employees as to those who remember the departed heroes personally.

The kind of "corporate culture" most appropriate for religious health care organizations has been well described in the book, *American Spirit—Visions of a New Corporate Culture,* by Lawrence M. Miller.[1] The author points out eight basic requirements:

1. A clear, well-understood, and thoroughly embraced mission that guides the activities of management as well as employees
2. An emphasis on consensus decision making in contrast to command or even consultative decisions
3. A constructive dissatisfaction with current performance and a constant striving for excellence
4. Sharing of both power and rewards by employees and management
5. Reward and recognition geared to demonstrated performance rather than position or tenure
6. Sufficient, appropriate, and timely information for both managers and employees to control and monitor performance
7. Organizational commitment to individual employees
8. Constant and consistent communications and actions devoted to long-term employee and customer well-being

The religious health care organization should have at least a head start in most of these requirements. It should have a clear, consistent, and meaningful mission; it should accord its employees a dignity and worth that promotes consensus decisions, sharing of power and rewards, and a lasting commitment to each employee. It should always strive toward excellence. Developing the information, performance evaluation, and reward systems consistent with such values should then come fairly easily.

Experience suggests that the quickest and perhaps the most effective way to move the organization in the desired direction is through the supervisors. By making them into managers who design and direct their own approaches to excellence rather than simply following the designs and directions of those above them, supervisors can promote living out the organization's commitments more effectively. Moreover, the organization's structure probably will become leaner and flatter, promoting better communications as well as efficiency.

My personal experience suggests that carrying the idea one step further and turning employees into supervisors works equally well. Such devices as marketing circles make employee groups into their own supervisors, thereby allowing their former supervisors to function as managers. By challenging employees, supervisors, and managers together to define who the organization is and to develop ways of demonstrating that identity in day-to-day relations with each other and with customers, the organization's commitments can be translated into reality.

In addition to these administrative suggestions for personalizing the organizations, specific operational steps have been used with great success. Hospitals, for example, have developed valet service parking for patients with mobility problems. Although parking lots may give favored locations to physicians, such valet service demonstrates a commitment to making the institution as accessible as possible to the patient, as well as showing how important each patient is. Some hospitals have offered valet service as part of VIP packages, but such discriminatory treatment is counter to commitments to the dignity and worth of each individual. It would be wiser to offer the service to all patients, knowing that those with no mobility or ego problems are likely to make it on their own.

Guide service for patients and visitors is another type of effective personal gesture that works. The access of religious health care organizations to volunteers helps in this regard. Providing personal assistance in negotiating the often confusing course of larger facilities is a clear manifestation of welcome as well as a demonstration of commitment. Managers and employees should be encouraged to fill in wherever volunteers are unavailable.

Assigning a specific personal nurse to each patient is another way to personalize the organization. The nurse should be as familiar with the patient's family and social situation as the physician, and as much the patient's champion as a technical professional. Introducing the hospital patient to the nurse on the next shift or whoever will take over the patient's care is a way of demonstrating a personal relationship. Calling hospital patients after discharge is another. In nursing homes, the longer length of stay demands as well as facilitates a lasting, personal relationship, but even there, each patient should have a satisfying relationship with a personal nurse.

In hospitals, personalization can begin with preadmission contact for scheduled admission patients. Having the admission representative establish a personal contact, make an appointment for completing the admission process, arrange for transport (even take the patient to the room in some cases), and make a postdischarge phone call to each such patient are ways of showing the hospital's personality. My personal preference calls for hospitality representatives to handle the entire process, including making visits to patients during their stay as personal representatives of administration. In effect, each patient has three specific persons as patient champions: the medical staff physician in charge, the primary nurse, and the hospitality representative. This last person has a different job description than a typical admissions clerk but focuses on starting the inpatient stay off right, then keeping it that way.

In nursing homes, the longer length of stay facilitates the use of resident champions. One individual may well be able to play the role for the entire institution, although having nurse's aides redesignated as resident aides is useful given the 24-hour, 7-days-a-week need for personal champions. With the infrequent presence of the personal physician, only two types of personal champion are available, nursing and hospitality, and the same person may serve both functions. Each resident and every family member should feel that they can go to one person who will see to any problem or need.

Another way to personalize an institution is to expect and enable each employee to know and greet each patient or resident by name. This means that housekeeping, dietary staff, technicians, and anyone else in contact with patients and residents will have to have easy access to the names of everyone they serve, by computer or paper as appropriate. In addition, both the employee and the institution must recognize that they *are* the organization. For casual, unexpected contacts when employees cannot be expected to know patient or resident names, they should still acknowledge and greet patients and visitors.

These are intended merely to illustrate the types of things religious health care organizations can do to establish a more personalized relationship with patients and residents. For further ideas, administrators, managers, and employees can think back on their own favorite bank, restaurant, hotel, airline, or other service experiences and pick out what made them special. In addition, each member of the organization should look for ideas in current and future encounters with such service organizations, many of whom are striving to personalize their customer relationships.

Administrators, managers, and employees should strive regularly and systematically, both individually and in groups, to think of ways they can personalize the organization and its relations with patients, residents, and other customers. Each intangible personal judgment dimension can be selected for separate attention. In addition, any change in procedure intended to enhance technical quality, productivity, or efficiency should be reviewed for potential effect on perceptions of intangible personal dimensions, as well as on institutional ones.

External Marketing Steps

In the description stage of marketing, the religious health care organization can promote personalization in various ways. First and foremost is to communicate both directly and indirectly about specific internal marketing steps taken: valet service, personal hospitality representatives, personal nurses, guide services, and so forth. The organization can simply describe the fact of such services and count on audiences reaching appropriate conclusions. Testimonials from past patients and residents can also be used, and should address both the specific steps taken and the conclusions the patients and residents reached about them.

The organization should strive to design and implement its marketing communication efforts on themes of personal identity. It should make every effort to think of itself not as a place or thing but as a person. The heroes who most closely demonstrate the organization's values and personality should be used in communications, just as they are used in internal marketing. Personal anecdotes as well as heroic acts should be used to give the public a sense that they know such heroes, even though they are long since departed. Many such heroes are likely to be clergy, sisters, or other persons linked to the specific religion that sponsors the organization. Their personal as much as their religious characteristics should be the focus of communication efforts aimed at making them widely known.

Communications about the organization should refer to it as "people" rather than a place or thing. Brochures about the hospital or nursing home can use pictures of people and treat information as direct communications from them. For example, physicians can be shown as the sources of descriptions of specific medical programs. Nurses can be shown as sources of information on nursing care, dieticians as sources on food, and housekeepers as sources on their services. Any service delivered in the institution is delivered by people. Showing them as the sources of information about such services will not only personalize the information to its intended audiences, but also will send a strong message to employees as well.

Advertisements can also use a personal approach. Trustees, administrators, managers, and employees can all serve as spokespersons in newspaper and magazine ads and TV and radio commercials. They may not be charismatic, but such persons can be credible and personal in speaking for their organizations. Using both managers and employees as spokespersons will also tend to strengthen their sense of ownership of the organization, as well as promote the efforts of other managers and employees in word-of-mouth communication.

Using members of the organization in marketing communications can also be part of the internal marketing approach. Appearing as a spokesperson is likely to be a significant honor to most people, even though appearing in a commercial and having to speak lines may create enormous stage fright for many. This honor may be part of a reward and recognition system used by management for those who have made significant contributions to personalizing the institution. Spokespersons might be selected by employees based on their sense of who the heroes are. This latter approach again can strengthen the employees' feeling that they own the organization.

Patients, residents, and other customers may be attracted to the idea of a partnership in their care. When this involves patients and family members in addition to care professionals, the personal approach to communication can show how such partnerships work. Here testimonials from prior experiences are better than the organization's own comments. Besides the outcomes of the care experience, patients, family members, and others should give their feelings and it should be featured in such communications.

Even the language of communication can be personalized. Instead of referring to the hospital or nursing home as an "it," the pronouns "we" and "our" can be employed. This will help in selecting more personal verbs, adjectives, and adverbs as well. This personalization should permeate all communications, including telephone and correspondence as well as publicity and advertising. News releases should always cite a spokesperson, for example, and use personal quotations wherever appropriate. Advertising should employ personal statements and show persons rather than places and things.

In many ways, health care organizations should take on the characteristics and "persona" of mothers: caring, comforting, warm, embracing, protecting, and nurturing. Health care institutions are at least surrogate parents caring for the needs of persons who are temporarily or perhaps permanently reduced to the status of a child as well as a customer. If religious health care organizations can think of themselves as indulgent rather than authoritarian parents and engage in some therapeutic pampering, they are likely to find the basis for communicating what kind of "persons" they are.

As with suggestions for internal marketing steps, these examples of external marketing steps are intended as illustrations rather than an exhaustive list of recommendations. As individual organizations decide who they are and what traits they wish to communicate to the public, they will probably think of many innovative approaches. The effect and effectiveness of such communication should be tested by asking the customers who will be affected. Pretesting of communications through focus group or other guided discussion should also include discussions by physicians and employees. Communications are commitments by the organization's members as well as messages to the public; thus they should be made with the full support of those who will have to fulfill the promises made.

Employing the suggestions discussed in Chapter 8 will enable the organization to use evidence of positive personal characteristics in its daily interactions with its customers as well as in its communications. Marketing through evidence will help religious health care organizations live out their values as well as promote their success. Health care consumers want and need religious providers to be the "persons" their values commit them to be. By consistently being and becoming widely known as the kind of persons the public want them to be, health care organizations enhance the quality of life of those they serve, as well as enhancing their likelihood of surviving.

Marketing concepts and techniques offer a unique way of identifying and responding to the needs of people. Marketing demands that we begin our efforts with those we serve, what they know, think, and feel. What we know, think, and feel comes next, and always in the context of the customer. With our commitments to service, religious health care organizations should not find marketing strange or uncomfortable, since we will use it to better serve the people we have set out to serve. Marketing only insists that we add to our own notions of what people need, their own perceptions of what they want and need.

There are no guarantees in marketing, any more than there are in health care. People are unpredictable and changeable; they require constant vigilance to keep up with their wants and whims as well as their enduring human needs. Marketing offers specific ways of discovering and responding to such wants, whims, and needs so that those who use it well can better serve the public and better ensure the success of their mission and their own survival. When religious health care organizations use marketing to ensure the living out of their values and responsiveness to the values of their customers, they will promote their success and survival, and well deserve both.

Footnotes

1. Miller, L. *American Spirit: Visions of a New Corporate Culture.* New York: Warner Books, 1984.

GLOSSARY

action - the cognitive script component that covers what patients and providers do during the care experience

advertising - marketing communication through paid public media

agenda-setting effect - the effect that marketing communications have on what people think about, judgment criteria they use

AIDA - awareness, interest, decision, action in a hierarchy of effects sequence

appropriation - the amount of money set aside for marketing or advertising purposes by an organization

argument - the set of persuasive logical statements that may support an assertion, as opposed to evidence

assertion - describing what is offered in subjective, judgmental terms, claiming distinctions or superiorities

association - communicating information without direct statements by linking services or providers with symbols or feelings

atmospherics - environmental, setting factors that influence patient attraction and satisfaction, especially by symbols

attribute set - the set of judgment dimensions or criteria that people use in determining preferences together with their perceptions of competing choices on such attributes

availability-valence model - communications effects based on what is most readily remembered and how valued it is

behavior-intention model - communications effects based on value times probability of personal consequences plus personal and social attitudes toward specific behavior

belief consistency - notion that claims or descriptions are inhibited or assisted in effect by what audience already believes

belief dynamics - theory of communication based on how existing beliefs affect what is read or heard, what impact occurs

body - the section of a message that provides explanation, evidence, or argument to support its theme

budget - the plan for allocating a marketing or advertising appropriation

campaign - an organized series of messages aimed at producing a specific mind-set position or marketing result

characters - the cognitive script component covering the people that participate in the care experience

clockwork - timing messages with rigid regularity

cluster analysis - a research/analytical tool for grouping respondents by similar facts or attitudes into segments

cognitive script - a model of the patient experience based on setting, props, characters, costumes, action, and dialogue *communication channel* - any method used to deliver a message, including personal contact, publicity, advertising, and word-of-mouth communication

communications positioning - a positioning strategy based on distinctiveness or superiority of communications

comparisons - messages that include comparative statements relative to competitors, named or unnamed

competition - all possible responses to a given problem or need other than the one intended

competitive positioning - a positioning strategy based on service distinctions or superiorities

confidence - how strongly beliefs are held by people in an audience as a result of communications

conjoint analysis - a research/analytical tool for identifying the critical attributes in program design

consumer decision model - a model of consumer choice in phases from problem recognition to background information to information search to evaluation to selection to implementation

convenience clinic - a source of episodic or regular medical or dental care emphasizing convenient hours, no need for appointments

concept testing - preliminary evaluation of a service program or communications idea through group discussion

consequences - the benefits and costs people expect from a given behavior or choice

context - the message/media setting, in what program commercial is aired, in what publication, story, section ad is placed

copy testing - prepublication evaluation of message content through group discussion or experimental exposure

costumes - the cognitive script component that covers what people wear and its effect on customer perceptions

credibility - attribute of message or of source of communication based on how believable each is

crescendo - timing messages so as to begin with infrequency, then increase in frequency toward saturation

customer - anyone whose choices and behavior in the market affect successs and survival

deception - using communications to mislead or misinform the audience to a significant degree

decision - the strategic and tactical planning phase of marketing between discovery and design

delivery - the internal operational phase of marketing between design and description

description - the communications phase of marketing between delivery and discovery

design - the program development and adjustment phase of marketing between decision and delivery

dialogue - the cognitive script component covering everything said to, by, and within the hearing of customers

differentiated communications - sending messages to more than one market or segment tailored to interests of each

differentiated marketing - designing and delivering services tailored to separate interests of markets or segments

direct delivery - sending messages directly to intended audiences via mail or delivery services

direct hook - a request for action in a message which asks for a contact with the sender

discovery - the research phase of marketing between description and decision

display advertising - placing messages where intended targets will see or find them

dissonance avoidance - the tendency of people to adopt perceptions and attitudes after the fact to justify preference and behavior

dynamics of communication - the way messages and campaigns affect the knowledge, attitudes, and behavior of audiences

effect evaluation - determining the total effects of communications and marketing efforts, and the value thereof

effectiveness - accomplishing what was intended for marketing and communications efforts

efficiency - accomplishing without wasting effort and expenditure

emotional content - message/copy content that aims at arousing emotions through words, sounds, or pictures

expectations - what people believe will occur during or as a result of a care experience

exposure - a single presentation of a message to an audience member, whether or not the member pays attention to it

facilitators - messages and actions that ease the way toward implementing preferences

factor analysis - research/analytical tool that identifies factors or underlying themes that organize groups of responses

factual distinctions - differences among services or providers that are objective, measurable, verifiable

fear appeals - messages and campaigns that motivate by citing negative consequences of not adopting intended behavior

features - objective, tangible aspects of service program or patient experience that produce intangible opinions

feedback - arranged comments by patients, employees, and others regarding their experiences during and after the fact *flighting* - sending messages in timed spurts during a campaign

focus groups - a structured, small group discussion of concepts, copy, programs, or strategies

focused communications - messages and campaigns aimed at the interest of a single market or segment

focused marketing - designing and delivering services and patient experiences aimed at a single market or segment

follower - a market or mindset position in the same category as the leader, but clearly behind

free association - a technique for determining mindset positions through open-ended questioning soliciting first impressions

frequency - the number of times an intended audience is exposed to a message

functional analysis - a research/analytical tool for identifying the tangible features most valued by customers

grabber - the sound, sight, or words used to gain attention to a message by an intended audience

guarantee - a promise intended to raise confidence in a claim or assertion

guest - a patient, family member, resident, client, or any other visitor to a health care provider or organization

halo effect - the tendency of people to improve their perceptions to reinforce their preferences, also the effect of one question and answer in a survey on answers to subsequent questions

health belief model - consumer decision process based on beliefs in seriousness of problem, susceptibility to them, likelihood of positive effect if action taken, cues to action

hierarchy of effects - communications create awareness, then specific knowledge, then opinions, attitudes, and behavior

hierarchy of needs - Maslow's notions of basic physical, security, belonging, esteem, and actualization needs

hook - a specific request for audience action in a message, whether direct or indirect

hyperbole - outrageously exaggerated statement or description, usually for humorous effect, usually about competition

image - the overall impression people have of a service or provider

image building - action and communication intended to reinforce or improve image rather than build utilization specifically

indirect hook - request for response to message that does not involve contacting the sender

information processing model - theory that communications create associations between service or provider and specific valued attributes without conscious audience involvement *inoculation* - beating the competition to the punch by conveying their news instead of waiting for them to do so

involvement - the level of interest or motivation present in the customer when considering and making a market decision

leader - a mindset or market position ahead of everyone else in a given category of responses

leverage - the amount of "business" or utilization that will result from achieving a top mindset position

life-style segment - a homogeneous set of customers who share common life styles: attitudes, interests, and behaviors

location - a place in the mind along judgment dimensions or in overall preference; the physical site of a service provider

logo - a visual or aural symbol associated with a service or provider

loyalty - strength of preference based on past use and satisfaction

market assessment - a systematic analysis of a real or potential market prior to deciding whether to enter it

market position - status of markets and shares therein associated with a given service or provider

market segment - a group of customers who can be treated as if they are alike within the group and significantly different from other groups in the same market

marketing - "the process of planning and executing the conception, pricing, promotion, and distribution of ideas, goods, and services to create exchanges that satisfy individual and organizational objectives" (according to the American Marketing Association)

marketing audit - a systematic analysis of current marketing efforts and success and the reasons therefor

marketing communications - any messages intended for marketing purposes

marketing intelligence - analyzed information about markets and competitors useful in making strategic and tactical decisions

marketing mix - the set of components used to pursue marketing objectives: product, place, price, and promotion

marketing plan - an organized set of action and communication intentions aimed at specified program success and its determinants

media - categories of paid ways to deliver messages, including newspapers, magazines, radio, and television

media plan - an organized set of choices regarding use of and expenditures for various media

mindset position - preference status and attribute perceptions associated with a given service or provider

mission - a statement of the basic business a provider is in, its reason for operating, whom it serves and how

multidimensional scaling - an analytical/presentation tool for showing where competing services and providers are positioned

name recognition - a measure of familiarity of competing services and providers

noise - confusing overabundance of messages reaching an audience

nominal groups - a technique for obtaining information about preferences from small groups

nonverbal content - message content not derived from words, includes tone of voice, body language, etc.

participant - someone other than the patient who plays a significant role in making a service or provider choice

patient promises - commitments to patients regarding their experience

peer preference - what other people want or expect them to do, as perceived by customers

perceptual mapping - identifying and portraying mindset positions along significant value dimensions

permanent display - messages that are "permanently" available to audiences through posters, directories, etc.

place - all aspects of the service operation that affect how convenient it is to obtain service, e.g., location, hours, etc.

point-of-purchase displays - messages displayed at the site of service, used to reinforce choice, promote other services or basic satisfaction

portfolio analysis - a way of examining individual "products" and markets based on market position and profitability

positioning - action and communications strategies focused on achieving and maintaining a desired mindset/market position

preference - relative ranking of competing options in terms of which is best for a given need

price - everything negative that customers have to endure, everything they "pay" in return for product benefits

probing - asking for additional answers or for reasons behind answers in interviews or surveys

product - the set of benefits that people expect and receive through a purchase/use experience

product line - a set of related services that addresses the same problem, serves the same market or segment, and can be marketed in a coordinated fashion

product-line marketing - marketing strategy and tactics organized around specific product lines

props - tools, equipment, items used by patients and providers during the care experience

prospect - any potential guest or customer

public - any group of individuals or organizations whose attitudes and behavior can help or hurt the organization

public service announcements - information on services or events that are transmitted free by public media

publicity - information transmitted by public media without charge, including news, features, notices, etc.

qualifier - part of a message, usually in the grabber, or part of a survey questionnaire used to ensure audiences and respondents are members of an intended market or segment

qualitative - covering attributes that can only be described through words, not numbers

quantitative - covering attributes that can be measured and described through numbers

reach - the number of people exposed to a given message

readership - the number of people who actually read a newspaper or magazine, as opposed to the number of subscribers; also the number of people who actually pay attention to a message, as opposed to the number exposed

recall - ability to remember a name or ad message when asked

recognition - ability to identify a message, sponsor, logo, etc. when prompted by seeing or hearing it

reference network - the people to whom customers turn for information or advice, or who otherwise influence customer choices

repetitions - successive transmissions of or exposures to the same message

repositioning - introducing new judgment criteria into customer evaluation and choice so as to improve mindset position

reputation - the overall state of esteem in which a service or provider is held by a market or segment

resistance - tendency of audiences to resist being persuaded by or even believing information counter to their beliefs

response - what people do when confronted with a problem, feeling a need, or as the result of a message

right brain/left brain - a model of cognitive/affective functioning used in evaluating message effects through brain wave measurements

risk reduction - a communications strategy based on reducing the risk potential customers feel in making the intended choice

sales promotion - offering free or discounted services or goods as short-time "specials" for new customers

saturation - flooding the media with messages to promote a specific service or event

scaling - a systematic way of assigning numbers to attitudes and feelings among customers *semantic differential* - a scaling approach based on verbal extremes

setting - location and all aspects of the service site or provider's facility that affect customer attraction and satisfaction

shopping - the tendency of customers to look at and try out alternative choices

signature - information in a message that identifies its sender and links the sender to the message content

significance - the meaning or symbolic value of a given behavior, service, or provider as perceived by customers and public

slogan - an easily remembered phrase that carries positive associations with a service or product

source effects - the impact that the source of a message has on its being attended, its credibility and impact

STARCH scores - standard measures of readership used in print media

subliminal communications - messages delivered in ways that only the unconscious mind perceives

targets - intended audiences for messages or the people to whom marketing efforts are directed

theme - the conclusion audiences are intended to reach as a result of a message experience

timing - the pattern of messages over time, e.g. saturation, crescendo, clockwork, flighting

top-of-mind - a place in the evoked set in which a service or provider comes first to mind, without any strong preference

trial behavior - people trying out a service or provider based on low-involvement interest rather than preference

trivial case - situation in which customers have low involvement and perceive little difference among competing choices; they tend to choose the most familiar

two-sided message - message that includes some negative information about sender, to add credibility or inoculate

values - what customers feel are important and worthy and thereby affect their attitudes and behavior

value dimensions - criteria customers use in judging competing choices

variability - tendency for people to differ significantly in their preferences, and to change their preferences over time

word-of-mouth - communications delivered by employees, patients, physicians, family members, and visitors that affect public impressions of services and providers, or advice given in response to requests that influences customer choices

Zeigarnik effect - tendency for people to complete unfinished slogans that are familiar to them

INDEX